The World's Worst Diabetes Mom

REAL-LIFE STORIES OF PARENTING A CHILD WITH TYPE 1 DIABETES

Stacey Simms

SPARK Publications
Charlotte, North Carolina

The World's Worst Diabetes Mom:
Real-Life Stories of Parenting a Child with Type 1 Diabetes
Stacey Simms

Designed, produced, and published by SPARK Publications, SPARKpublications.com
Charlotte, North Carolina

Portions of the author's previously published material have been reprinted with permission from the publishers of DiabetesMine.com and the book "Kids First, Diabetes Second."

Printed in the United States of America.
Softcover, October 2019, ISBN: 978-1-943070-66-4
E-book, October 2019, ISBN: 978-1-943070-67-1
Library of Congress Control Number: 2019910981

Dedication

For my mother, Arlene Simms, who never demanded perfection, but who always made sure I was safe and happy. I guess that makes you "worst" first.

For Slade, Lea, and Benny who fill my heart with laughter and love.

Medical Disclaimer

The information contained in this book is not intended as medical advice and is not a substitute for the services of and information from a trained health care provider.

Table of Contents

Introduction

This isn't the book I set out to write. The original idea was to put together a bunch of my old blog posts, add some updated information, and send it out into the world. But I found myself adding and rewriting and being frustrated with "just" the information. I've been a diabetes parent for more than 12 years. What did I really want to say?

Information is available in many places. You can Google any question you have right now. And a bunch of wonderful, informative diabetes books are already on the market. But I wanted to get to the bottom of what I'd learned after more than a decade of raising a child with type 1 diabetes (T1D) and more than four years hosting "Diabetes Connections," a podcast about T1D. How could I really add to the conversation and help?

Then someone on Facebook told me I was an awful parent.

Perfection has never sat well with me. It's also never sat close to me. With or without diabetes. My philosophy (and you'll hear it a lot in these pages) is "not perfect, but safe and happy." I was called out on that by another parent who vehemently disagreed. It got ugly, as can happen on social media, and I decided to back off. I gave up arguing and wrote, "I guess I'm the world's worst diabetes mom." That's when the lightbulb went on.

Our son was diagnosed in 2006, just before he turned 2 years old. Our diabetes philosophy has always been about acknowledging the bad and being realistic about how diabetes can mess things up and slow us down. We're not a "T1D will never stop us" kind of family. Diabetes stinks. It *can* stop you. But then you correct or treat or whatever you need to do to keep going and help your child live the life he or she wants. You cry, you laugh, and you keep moving forward.

Our endocrinologist, Dr. V, gave us a gift the first day we met him. In addition to getting down on the floor and playing with my son, Benny (and answering all of my questions – I basically gave him the equivalent of a job interview), he said that we needed to realize that a lot of treating and managing diabetes was as much of an art as a science. Over the next few months as we learned how to take care of Benny, Dr. V would help us see that numbers, while extremely important, weren't always exact and shouldn't be allowed to run our lives. He wanted Benny to grow up as a person with diabetes, not as a person defined by diabetes.

We needed to remember, always, that we were raising a child. Not a number, not a graph, not a lab result. Benny would always be more than his A1C or his time in range.

When I found the diabetes online community a few years later, I found not everyone was as lucky to have had that guidance early on. It also seemed like the worry about numbers, the search for exact measurements, and the pursuit of perfection were cropping up more and more. Since Benny's diagnosis in 2006, I've felt a shift from people talking and sharing about living well with type 1 diabetes to living perfectly with it.

Was this part of the trend in parenting where we all felt like we must be perfect to be successful and raise good kids? Is it unique to diabetes where we really do feel like we're graded on our actions? I mean, there are numbers every single day and, now with continuous glucose monitoring, every single minute. It's almost impossible to not correlate a feeling to those numbers.

I realized pretty quickly that I can't play that game. Perfection is not in my parenting wheelhouse. In fact, I welcome mistakes. It's how I learn. I improve by getting it wrong the first time around. I'd argue that mistakes make us all better.

Maybe you're just starting out with a newly diagnosed child. If so, I hope this book can guide you through some basic concepts and help you recognize that, while you will make mistakes, your child with diabetes can be safe and happy. If you've been in the diabetes community for a while, maybe instead of worrying about falling short, you'll see yourself in some of my stories. Either way, I want you to join me in deciding that there's a way to turn mistakes and missteps into your secret superpower.

Before we really dive in, and I reveal all my mistakes and embarrassing moments, it's important that I give a sort of baseline. Let there be no misunderstanding: We take diabetes and Benny's diabetes management and health very seriously. We are vigilant and very involved. I don't share A1Cs or other very personal health information, but Dr. V says Benny is right where he wants him to be.

We have never been back to the hospital (knock on wood) for anything diabetes related since diagnosis. In terms of tech, Benny has been on an insulin pump since age 2 (about six months after diagnosis) and has worn a continuous glucose monitor (CGM) since 2013, just a few days before he turned 9. My parenting goals, with and without diabetes, are to raise my children to be confident, independent and responsible.

This is not a book that will tell you how to eat or how to dose. I'm not a doctor, and this isn't a medical guide. It's not a guide to diabetes technology or advice about which type you should use and why. Rather, it's a look into our lives over the past 12 years of type 1 diabetes. Our journey so far has been full of challenges, stress, some mistakes, and lots of learning. But it's also been full of laughter, love, and joy.

If you are brand new to T1D, here's something else to keep in mind. Learning about diabetes is like drinking from a fire hose; the amount of information is impossible to take in all at once. The metaphor I like best came from our endocrinologist during those first overwhelming weeks. Type 1 diabetes is like you've woken up one morning to find your smooth drive to work suddenly full of red lights and construction. You can still get there, but it takes a lot more effort, time, and patience. Over a few weeks and months, the traffic thins out, the construction goes away, and you hit fewer red lights. But the commute itself is never the same. You take detours. You hit potholes. But you become a better driver than you ever imagined. Your reflexes improve, you enjoy the view, and you sing along to the radio.

It gets better. Really.

Even if you're The World's Worst Diabetes Mom.

CHAPTER 1

The Diagnosis

In the middle of October, he sent me a wild text. Seems that Benny had wet his crib overnight, but there was so much urine that it went through the mattress. "You won't believe the amount of pee that came out of this kid!" Slade wrote. I texted something back along the lines of, "Too bad it happened on your shift, haha!" We didn't think much of it, and after Slade did some laundry, we all went on with our day.

"You need to get your son to the hospital right now." The voice on the other end of the phone was shaky.

I looked over at my almost 2-year-old. Hospital? Surely that was a mistake. Benny hadn't been feeling well the day before – OK, he hadn't been feeling well for a few weeks – but he was playing and happy now. It was sunny! How could something bad happen on such a beautiful Saturday?

"Stacey, please listen. His blood sugar is extremely high, and you need to pack a bag and head down to the hospital. They're expecting you, and you'll be there for a few days."

If you're reading this, if you've picked up this book, you likely know the rest of our story. The confused rush of packing a bag, debating whether to bring our older child. The taking-forever ride to the hospital 45 minutes away. The news that all of our lives would change in ways we couldn't imagine.

"Your son has type 1 diabetes."

Like many families who hear those words, we started seeing the signs a few weeks prior.

My husband, Slade, and I worked opposite shifts at the time. I was a morning radio show host with a workday that started at 4 a.m. I left the house around 3:15 a.m. Slade owned and managed a restaurant, so his day started and ended much later. We split the child care, and while we didn't see each other very much during that time, we did very well with the kids.

Every day, Slade would text me with a morning update during the 7 a.m. news, when I had a quick break. Usually this was a funny picture or video of the kids, a short morning report, or just a "we're off to day care" message.

In the middle of October, he sent me a wild text. Seems that Benny had wet his crib overnight, but there was so much urine that it went through the mattress. "You won't believe the amount of pee that came out of this kid!" Slade wrote. I texted something back along the lines of, "Too bad it happened on your shift, haha!" We didn't think much of it, and after Slade did some laundry, we all went on with our day.

About a month later, I noticed Benny's personality was changing. He had been a happy, goofy kid since day one, but suddenly, he was cranky, tired, and irritable. He was drinking a lot more water and milk; it was getting hard to keep him in a dry diaper.

Thanksgiving was strange. One hour Benny was feeling fine and having fun with his cousins and grandparents. The next hour he'd just want to lie down and didn't want to play or even move around much. We knew something was wrong with our baby.

I called our pediatrician the Monday after Thanksgiving. Along with the morning radio show, I'd been a local TV news reporter specializing in health and medical news. I knew just enough about the symptoms of type 1 diabetes to ask about it.

Our doctor said she'd never seen anyone under age 2 with T1D but that we should bring him in so that they could rule it out.

Quick note: This was in 2006 when there really were fewer cases of babies with T1D. This was a large pediatric practice with hundreds if not thousands of children as patients. But Benny was the first child under the age of 2 to be diagnosed by this doctor. For years after, when we came in for regular checkups, the nurses and docs would check our chart and be amazed that he was diagnosed so young. They all knew him and were happy to see him growing and healthy.

That week, though, was very, very strange. A fasting glucose finger prick test Monday morning came back with a blood glucose (BG) of 80. They did a blood draw and a urine test. We got the results of the urine test pretty quickly. Of course, there was sugar in it. For some reason – and the story gets fuzzy here for me – we didn't get the blood draw/A1C results for days.

No one mentioned type 1 diabetes. I think the "normal" BG value threw them off. They treated Benny for a urinary tract infection, and by Wednesday he was feeling much better. His personality and behavior had improved (of course, that infection was probably painful!), but he was still drinking and peeing a ton.

I started surfing the internet. I was getting convinced that he had some rare kidney disease or bizarre infection. I started getting really scared. That's when the phone rang with the woman telling me to get to the hospital. The A1C test had come back, and while she didn't use those terms with us or tell me that number over the phone, she did say Benny's blood sugar was likely over 600 at that very moment and that we needed to get him to the children's hospital as soon as we could.

We stayed in that hospital for three days, learning to give shots, do fingersticks, and count carbs, and realizing things would never be the same again. Our 23-month-old son and just turned 5-year-old daughter were thrust into a new world where their parents were worried, and life was upside down. I cried – just once in front of my son – and buckets where he couldn't see me. Part of me was relieved because Benny had been sick for a while and at least now we had an answer; I could stop surfing the internet looking for the worst. I knew just enough about type 1, however, to know that our life was going to completely change.

In addition to my 10-plus years as a health reporter at that time, my radio station was the media sponsor for the local JDRF golf tournament. Every year, I'd interviewed families touched by T1D and talked to many kids living happily with it.

One little boy, Evan, told me he ate Pop-Tarts! Not every day, his mother added, rolling her eyes at him. Twins Maddie and Ashley were usually laughing and having fun. Thinking about those children and their families helped remind me that it was going to be OK, even before we began our education in the hospital.

A nurse poked her head in and introduced herself. Diagnosed with type 1 as a child, she made a point of visiting newly diagnosed families. She was also a mom and was pregnant! Seeing a happy, healthy adult with type 1 gave me so much hope and reassurance. She laughed and understood; it's why she tried to visit the newly diagnosed families.

After a whirlwind of instruction, shots, math, and doctors, they sent us home. Sent us home by ourselves with a handful of books and a bunch of medical stuff we didn't know existed a few days prior. Insulin vials, syringes, test strips, meters, ketone strips ... it was overwhelming to look at my toddler and realize we had to do *all this stuff.*

At the time, there was no easy way to find others with whom we could connect. Facebook was just dipping its toes beyond college students, Twitter was a few months old, and blogging was in its infancy. The iPhone wasn't even released until 2007. Even with my local radio station "connections" I felt very much alone.

I made mistakes. A lot of them. I poked myself with needles and lancets. I messed up injections (he wiggled!), and I messed up measuring. Of course, we got better ... well, until the next mistake. (Continue on, dear reader!)

And over the years, slowly and with a lot of work, I found what I needed more than anything. I found my community. This book isn't really about that, but anyone who knows me or has listened to the podcast or heard me speak knows that my passion is in-person connection. I started a dinner meet-up with other moms. I grew a local T1D parenting Facebook group to more than 700 members.

I started blogging about our journey just a month after Benny's diagnosis. My radio listeners wanted to know more, but our show wasn't formatted for personal stories. News, weather, traffic, and politics were our bread and butter. After a while, I realized the blog was much more for me than for anyone else. I never tried to reach a big audience. But recently, I've been hearing more and more from parents who say those older blog entries are helping – with school, day care, camp, and all the other issues our kids with T1D face. Because of that, I'm including a lot of blog entries in this book. Here's the very first post:

[FRIDAY, JANUARY 12, 2007]
Thank you!
Where do I start? It must be with thanks.
Thank you to everyone who emailed or called after I shared the news last month that my son's been diagnosed with type 1 diabetes. They used to call it juvenile diabetes, and it doesn't get more juvenile than Benny. The doctors gave us the news December 2nd, just one month shy of his 2nd birthday. It means his pancreas doesn't work and never will. His body doesn't make insulin, and he needs injections to stay alive.
Thank you to the incredible doctors and nurses at Carolinas Medical Center – especially our overnight nurse who also has type 1 diabetes. I can't tell you how much it meant to me that first night just to meet a successful, healthy, adult living with type 1. (And she's a mom! And she's expecting!)

Thanks to our pediatric endocrinologist, Dr. V, who made me feel perfectly normal every time I called him with another question. When you've never ever given a shot and suddenly your 2-year-old needs four or five a day, trust me, there's a lot to ask. *He moved! Did he get all the insulin? I pricked my finger (again)! I may have mixed up the long-acting and short-acting insulin vials! No wait, I didn't. Will Tylenol make his blood sugar go up? Does running around and falling down laughing, as only a 2-year-old can, bring his blood sugar down?* I love Dr. V. He has patience and a sense of humor (he needs both to deal with me), and he's a great doctor.

Thanks to my amazing husband, Slade. When we got home from the hospital, he threw open the cupboards and sprang into action. He set up "diabetes central" with all our supplies, everything organized, in our kitchen. We have a chart now that shows the carb count of all our kids' favorite foods. Pizza goldfish? Fifteen carbs per 40 fishes. Three-cheese tortellini? Thirty-three grams in 19. String cheese? Less than one carb per. Slade's set up a whole system to keep track of Benny's food, blood sugar, his shots. My Excel hero.

Thanks to my friends at WBT who didn't blink when I needed some time off. To my cohost Al Gardner who came over to play with Lea and Benny. And only sportscaster Jim Szoke could make me laugh about the challenge of holiday parties by making it sound as if I threw myself onto the cupcakes like they were grenades.

Thank you to every parent of a child with diabetes who emailed me to tell me that while things will never be the same, we will be OK. Thank you to all the grown-ups diagnosed with type 1 as kids who shared stories of how far treatment has come.

This blog will be a place to talk about my family's experience with diabetes, but also, I hope, a chance to share a little bit more about myself. Let me know what you think.

ASK YOUR DOCTOR

- What is the on-call number for urgent questions? Is there a separate number for non-urgent questions?

- Can you help us navigate insurance and/or diabetes supply questions? Do you know of a local resource that can?

- Why do you recommend the particular regimen and insulin type you're prescribing for my child? (Note: Insulin type may be dictated by your insurance.)

- Can you connect me with our local type 1 diabetes community?

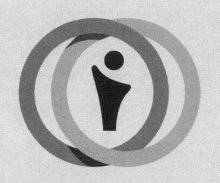

CHAPTER 2

The First
Night Home

How was I supposed to do a shot through the crib slats without waking him up? Forget this. I started to walk out of the room. You read that right. Our very first night home with diabetes, and I decided that we didn't have to deal with it. He'd be fine! It was worse to wake up a sleeping baby, right?

When you're giving a sleeping toddler an insulin shot, is it better to raise the crib rails or try to line up your aim and deliver the shot through the slats? This is not something they covered at the hospital.

We were sent home with pretty standard orders for a newly diagnosed child. We were to check BG around 11 p.m., then again overnight, and then around 6 a.m. In those days, I woke up for work around 2:30 a.m., so that turned out to be a good time for those overnight checks. It became pretty routine, but it started off as anything but.

Benny wasn't yet 2, and he was still sleeping in a crib. We were planning to transition him into a "big boy" bed sometime before he turned 3. We'd done the same thing with his sister, and it went fine. We were lucky not to have any climbers or jail-break babies.

Lea and Benny could be wild in other ways, but they slept in their cribs and later in their beds just fine.

We didn't anticipate any issues with diabetes and the crib. What that really means is that we didn't think about the crib at all until the first night we were back home. I walked into his room, ready to do a fingerstick and follow doctor's orders for the results.

Then I saw the slats.

What had seemed like an ordinary wooden crib suddenly looked like an impenetrable fortress. I was supposed to juggle a flashlight, a lancer, and a meter to check my child's teeny-tiny finger. I thought I was prepared for that. Now I was supposed to figure out a way to do it with Benny encased in what was basically a raised wooden box.

I'm pretty short, so going over the crib rail didn't seem like an option. Pulling it down seemed like a sure way to make a huge noise and wake up Mr. Excitement. You know that thing when your sleepy toddler wakes up and decides it's time to party? No, thank you.

Benny's hand was near the side of the crib, so I decided to chance reaching through the slats. Success! He was 255. I had done it! Benny was still asleep, and I had an actual number on the meter! My heart surged with pride. Best. Diabetes. Mom. Ever!

Just as quickly, my heart sank – 255? Our endocrinologist had advised giving a correction at that number. *Noooo!* I had completed the fingerstick without waking him up! How was I supposed to do a shot through the slats without a ruckus? Forget this. I started to walk out of the room.

You read that right. Our very first night home with diabetes, and I decided that we didn't have to deal with it. He'd be fine! It was worse to wake up a sleeping baby, right?

I faced a lot of decisions like this the first few weeks with Benny. So much of it was unpleasant. Our endo had urged us to be impassionate, to start right in with a routine and make diabetes as much of Benny's daily life as brushing his teeth and putting on shoes before he went outside. I recognized the wisdom in that advice; we didn't want to get into a position where we were giving him prizes and buying him ponies for every fingerstick and every shot.

But there were times when I thought, "Would a pony really be that bad?"

Our first two weeks with diabetes were rough. There is just no good way to communicate to a toddler that his pancreas is no longer working and that the shots and the pokes are going to make him feel better. He went from a needle-free life to the people he loved most trying to stab him all the time.

He adjusted to finger pricks easiest. He often didn't want to stop what he was doing, so we'd bring the kit to him and try to be quick. We found out he's ambidextrous, which is helpful. We also found that he liked to see just how much blood he could squeeze out and wipe all over the floor or table after we turned away. Not so helpful.

We did have to hold him for the first two weeks of shots. It was usually more of hug or a firm cuddle, but sometimes it was just flat-out wrestling down a crying, struggling 2-year-old. That was the worst. I'm feeling anxious again just typing this. I tried hard to be matter-of-fact, as our endo had suggested, and I do think it helped us all adjust. Sort of fake it till you make it. But of course, once Benny was asleep or I had time alone, I would let the tears flow.

A few people told us to look into shot blockers or other pain relief items. But others with type 1 told us the shots and fingersticks were just something to get used to. This is a really tough and individual decision. Ultimately, we decided if Benny didn't get used to things within a month or two that we'd seek other help or products.

I've heard good reviews about two retail products: Shot Blocker and Buzzy. They both work on the idea that distraction can reduce pain. Shot blocker is a small, U-shaped plastic piece with round bumps on the bottom. You press it gently into the skin, and the brain focuses on that sensation while you inject.

The Buzzy uses vibration and an ice pack to achieve similar results, and it's packaged to look like a cute little bumblebee.

Years later, long after we'd switched from multiple daily injections (MDI) to a pump, I found out about some other options. There are two products I know of: the I-Port Advance injection port and the Insuflon port. Very similar to the way a pump inset connects to the body, these go in with a needle and leave behind a small cannula under the skin and a raised piece above the skin. It's held on by adhesive and stays in place for three days, during which time you can give insulin injections without piercing the skin again. The bad news is that, as of this writing, very few insurance companies cover the cost of these devices.

When Benny was much older and started doing his own shots and inset placements, I read a study that coughing during injections alleviated pain. This actually worked for him! I can now tell when Benny is doing a site change – even if I'm not in the room – because I hear an exaggerated loud cough. Not recommended for when someone else is doing the site or the injection – too easy for the person coughing to move or jerk suddenly and create an issue.

Even without extra pain-relief efforts, our situation did improve and actually started feeling like a routine, just like Dr. V said it would. I was surprised how quickly that happened. After those first two weeks, as long as he didn't have to stop playing for very long, he would just hold up his arm or stick out his leg. We got quick and discreet – I once gave Benny a shot while sitting in the audience at a kids' theater show. He didn't want to get up and miss anything, so we stayed put. I'm not sure anyone around us even noticed. After only a few weeks, we'd actually gotten pretty good at this shot stuff!

But back at that first night home, as I started to sneak out of his room, "pretty good" seemed a very long way off. I was still holding the meter case in my hand when I got to the door and almost stepped out into the hallway. But there, in the dark quiet, it hit me.

Diabetes wasn't going anywhere. There was no room for magical thinking. This was about Benny's health and what he needed, not about my reluctance. If he woke up, so be it. My fear wasn't really about disrupting his sleep schedule anyway.

You see, giving him the shot that first night meant this was real, that it had followed us home, that diabetes was in my house, that it was in his crib. Acknowledging that wasn't something I wanted to do. But Benny needed us to stand with him, not sneak off and wish diabetes away.

I took a deep breath. I needed to get it together. *Snap out of it, Mom, and go give him that shot.* So I did.

You remember those first few times, right? There are a few steps after you prime and dial up the pen or draw up the insulin. I pinched up the skin, injected slowly, and counted to five to make sure all the insulin went in. We were using teeny-tiny doses at the time, so we had to use a syringe, no pen to measure down to the quarter units we were using.

I don't remember if Benny woke up, but I do remember an amazing feeling of triumph. I did it! I wanted to shout it out and high-five someone! If social media had been around, you know there would have been some serious posting: #NighttimeNinja, #DMomGetsItDone or something like that.

Instead, I went back to my room and got back into bed. I remember thinking, very logically, that through the crib slats was the right way to go, even with shots. I did all the finger pokes and injections that way overnight until Benny moved into a bed. He was closer to 3 by then, just as we'd planned, and it was a great day. We even chose blue and red sheets and blankets, so the blood drops wouldn't show.

They also didn't cover that at the hospital.

ASK YOUR DOCTOR

- What is my child's blood glucose range during the day and overnight? (This can vary greatly, especially among the newly diagnosed and very young children.)

- What do I need to know about best practice with pens or syringes?

- What's the best way to rotate injection sites, and why is that important?

- Is a shot blocker device or something like I-Port Advance a good option? (Also check your insurance coverage on these devices.)

CHAPTER 3

Life Goes On

I called my mother and told her the trip was off.
"That's ridiculous," she said. "Life goes on. You
have to go!" I hadn't even thought that was an
option. How could life go on like that? I had still had
a lot of questions every day. It felt like the learning
curve was always going to stay steep. Besides, what
kind of mother leaves her newly diagnosed kiddo
with type 1 behind while she goes and gambles in
the desert? Apparently, this one.

I joke that in the first month of diabetes I called our
endocrinology office every single day. The secret about that is,
it's not a joke. I really did call that often.

Usually it was for a question about dosing or logging or
counting carbs or making judgment calls for a toddler who's
getting wisps of insulin drawn up in a syringe not designed for
teeny-tiny doses. But sometimes it was because I'd stabbed myself
with the needle meant for Benny.

I also called when I got insulin in my mouth (it was on my
hand when I wiped my lips), when I wasn't sure if I'd really
given a shot, and for many other mishaps. I vividly remember
trying Benny's tummy for an injection site. I pushed the needle
in and squirted myself with insulin! I don't know how I did it,

but the needle hadn't actually gone under the skin, I had poked it through his skin and out the other side *like a sewing needle.* Benny laughed. I promise you, my not-yet-2-year-old saw me squirt myself with insulin with a needle sticking out of his stomach, and he laughed at me. Hoo boy.

Despite my mistakes, we stumbled through without any emergencies or dire situations. I was almost feeling like I could handle things. That lasted about three weeks.

Then we went to Wannado City.

Wannado City was an indoor role-playing amusement park. It's closed now, but it was a cute concept. Your child could be a firefighter, a fashion model, lawyer, TV reporter, whatever they wanted to do. (Get it? Whatever they *wanna do*). They were issued make-believe bank accounts and fake money and went from store to store pretending to do lots of grown-up stuff.

This was part of a long-planned trip to visit my parents just three weeks after Benny's diagnosis. They live in Florida (we're in North Carolina), so we started thinking about how diabetes would travel. I wasn't too worried. Our doctor had said just to double-check our supplies, and my parents live close to healthcare and pharmacies. Plus, we'd all be together.

It would be the first time we'd seen my mom and dad, my sister, and her family since T1D entered our lives. I remember walking into my parents' home, determined to show them that we knew what we were doing, that they didn't need to worry, and that we had diabetes under control.

That lasted about five minutes. Then I burst into tears. I'm very close to my mother and sister. There was no way I would be able to cover it up. It makes me laugh now to think that I could! I was holding in a lot of emotion, a lot of pressure. It actually felt great to get it out.

We all went to Wannado City a few days into the trip. We got there in the morning, had lunch and counted carbs thanks to the CalorieKing book – remember that we had no smart phones at this time. About an hour later, we watched Benny play with his older cousins and sister and wondered if we'd be able to get him down for a nap.

Suddenly, Benny stumbled. Well, there you go, we said, he obviously needs to sleep. I picked him up, and we brought over the stroller. Slade wanted to check Benny, but I was reluctant because he was already closing his eyes, and I didn't want to wake him up. But we were trying to be good and keep to our new diabetes schedule, so we checked him.

He was 32. I'm pretty sure that sleepy kid I was holding wasn't napping; he was passing out.

All I had left in my diaper bag was a fruit roll-up and glucose tabs. No way were we going to get him to chew and swallow. Slade ran over to a snack stand and grabbed a bottle of juice. Luckily, Benny was awake enough to drink it, and he quickly swallowed it down.

This was our very first time with a scary low. We made sure my mom could take care of our daughter, and we left Wannado City with Benny. We just picked up and took off. I couldn't imagine any other scenario. Surely we'd need to do something else to help him recover. I called our doctor who reassured us he'd be fine, to just test frequently and take it easy the rest of day.

Benny wanted to eat right away (our first experience with low-sugar hunger), and soon he was happily munching on some snacks.

I'll never forget turning around and looking at my 23-month old, strapped into his car seat, happy as can be for that ride home. I was amazed at the power of the low to take him down and then the power of simple sugar to bring him back. Our emergency supplies were going to be juice and candy? It seemed absurd. After all this time, I'm still amazed at the power of sugar – it's our best friend and worst enemy.

The rest of our trip to Florida was less eventful, although I do remember Benny wiping his fingers on my mother's beautiful floor after a BG check and chasing his sister around with the blood on the end of his finger. So basically normal toddler T1D stuff.

We'd made it through our first trip after diagnosis, but we had another vacation coming up. In late January, almost exactly two months after Benny's diagnosis, Slade and I were supposed to go to Las Vegas with my college roommate and her husband. That trip had been a long time in the planning, and we were all really looking forward to it.

Of course, we had to cancel.

I called my mother – who was set to come up and stay with the kids – and told her the trip was off.

"That's ridiculous," she said. "Life goes on. You have to go!"

I hadn't even thought that was an option. How could life go on like that? I mean, sure, Benny was back to feeling great, eating well, and adjusting to the pokes and shots. We were starting to settle into something like a routine, but I still had a lot of questions every day. It felt like the learning curve was always going to stay steep. Besides, what kind of mother leaves her newly diagnosed kiddo with type 1 behind while she goes and gambles in the desert? Apparently, this one.

It took a lot of planning. And worrying. But I took my mother's words to heart. Life did need to go on, and we were fortunate to have caregivers willing to learn and look after my son.

But wait! I left out the best part! Right after my mother gifted me with that terrific life philosophy, she added this: "You should go. But I don't think I can give him shots."

I remember feeling so inspired by her can-do attitude and then bursting out laughing. Of course he had to have insulin shots while we were away! Aw, Mom.

I often say that we are the luckiest family I know when it comes to type 1. And this story really bears that out. Both of my kids were in day care, and their caregivers really did go above and beyond. The day care manager had some medical experience and was one of the most caring, open-hearted women I've ever met. Even better, they already had a little girl with diabetes there. Her mother, a teacher, had created a guide and taught the staff many of the basics. Another care provider was also in nursing school, and she stepped up quickly to assist and give Benny his shots. It was amazing.

We called the nursing student and asked if she was willing to come over and give Benny the shots he needed throughout the weekend. She saved the day and did it. Of course, we paid her, but how about that?

We planned for Vegas as best we could and then took off for a long weekend of catching up, eating too much, and trying to have fun. I was worried and checked in a ton, but my mother promised she'd keep me posted, and I tried to relax. It worked, mostly. There was one time that my phone rang as I was getting into an elevator at the Aladdin hotel (now demolished, not my fault). It was about midnight back home, and my mother was worried about a high blood sugar. Of course, as soon as the elevator doors closed, the call cut off.

As I fretted in Vegas, my mother dialed up the endo on call. The head of the practice was answering the phone that night, and my mom and Dr. P had a great conversation that she still refers to today, more than 12 years later. He told her that one high blood sugar is fixable and not something to lose too much sleep over. He talked to her about lows and at what point she should be worried and when to treat as calmly as a grandma can. Dr. P really put her mind at ease.

He also told her to check ketones. Ketones are acids that build up when your body starts to burn fat for energy. They indicate that you need more insulin. Ketones can build up with high blood sugar, but they can also come on during illness or other circumstance. You usually need insulin and water to flush them out.

You can use urine strips or a blood ketone meter to check. Some people are more prone to ketones than others, and we were told that most levels of ketones below large on a test strip or below 1.5 on a blood ketone meter can be managed at home, as long as the person can swallow fluids. This is a definite "talk to your doctor" situation because a significant buildup of ketones can lead to DKA, diabetic ketoacidosis, a very serious condition that can lead to coma or even death.

We didn't have a blood ketone meter at the time, and Benny was still in diapers. How do you get a kid who isn't potty trained to pee on a stick? Let me know if you figure that one out. In the hospital, they had placed cotton balls in his diaper and then squeezed them out onto the ketone stick. Gross but effective. Mom still talks about that too. No ketones. So no need for more cotton balls that night.

When she was able to reconnect with me, everything was under control. The weekend wasn't perfect, but Benny was safe and happy. My mother had new confidence, and she knew we had great health care providers. I think knowing that I could call that doctor anytime went a long way in easing her mind.

Looking back, I'm so glad we went. I don't remember too much of the trip itself – I'm sure we lost some money and gained some weight – but it stands out as how we set the tone for our lives with diabetes. Taking that trip taught me that life really does go on.

My parenting style has always been teaching independence to my kids and being excited at the idea of them being strong and smart enough to be on their own. I had to be reminded that I deserve the same. And it's no mistake that my mother is the one who reminded me.

ASK YOUR DOCTOR

- What's the on-call number, and when should I use it?

- What do I need to know about ketones? What ketone measurement device do you recommend? (Also check with your insurance company about what's covered.)

- At my child's age, what would you recommend caregivers need to know? Can you help me make a list of top priorities?

CHAPTER 4

Pump Start

I checked everywhere. No cartridge. No special
needle. That meant no way to put more insulin
into the pump. That meant no more pump. I won't
tell you who packed all the diabetes supplies, but
his name rhymes with *played*, as in *played golf
in Vermont* while I was freaking out in New York.
Even with Slade away, I knew we'd be safe; we
could switch back to shots. But first, I wanted to try
everything I could to keep Benny pumping. We had
just started!

I began our research on insulin pumps soon after Benny was
diagnosed. It's really not that long ago, but in 2007 many
endocrinologists still thought it was a bad idea to prescribe an
insulin pump for a toddler. We felt strongly that Benny would
benefit from the precise dosing and flexibility that pumping
offers. Luckily, our endo agreed. As is typical, our insurance
company made us wait about six months after diagnosis, and our
endo encouraged us to use that time to really learn the basics
of diabetes.

In recent years, I've seen many people jump into an insulin
pump and CGM much more quickly. That's fine, but in my
opinion, it's smart to learn the basics of diabetes first. All tech can

fail. We need to be comfortable with and knowledgeable about shots and fingersticks.

We've also found that really knowing how to dose and understanding how your individual child's body reacts can help you take advantage of all the pumps have to offer. For some, that takes two weeks. For others, it may take two years or even longer. You don't want to be stuck with a pump problem at 2 a.m. and not know your child's correction factor, or have to call your JDRF chapter to ask them to walk you through a fingerstick because the CGM isn't working. I heard you laugh just now, but I didn't make that up. I know the JDRF staffer who took that call.

Before I share our pump start stories, let's go through some basics. Please keep in mind that these are my observations as a layperson. Talk to your educator or endocrinologist about insulin pumps and any other diabetes gear before making any decisions.

There are two main types of insulin pumps: tubed and tubeless. Both are small mechanical devices a little larger than a pager, worn outside the body. Both deliver insulin through a small cannula under the skin, and that cannula is inserted with a needle. In most cases, the needle goes in then comes out and leaves the cannula behind, a few millimeters below the skin.

A tubed pump can have auto-inserters or, for the very brave, manual inserters, which means exactly what it sounds like – you push the needle in by hand. As I mentioned, most inserters leave a plastic cannula under the skin, but steel needle infusion sets actually leave a tiny needle. They're recommended more for people with scarring, reactions to plastic or other issues. All infusion sets stay in place for two to three days, and then you insert a new one in a new location. The pump delivers the insulin through a thin, flexible, plastic tube – anywhere from 24 to 48 inches long – that attaches to the infusion set.

Benny has always worn a tubed pump. We started with Animas 2020 in July 2007, switched to the Animas Ping in 2011 and now use the Tandem t:slim X2.

You can wear a tubed pump anywhere on the body, and with

all pumps, you must rotate sites. Benny's favorite spot is his stomach, just above his belt line, and he puts the pump in his pocket. For the first 10 years, he had a little pouch on his belt. I've seen people wear tubed pumps on their arms, in special shirt pockets, in bras, on their legs, and even on backs and chests. This is a pretty creative community!

The tubeless pump is generally referred to as a "pod" because the brand name is Omnipod. With this type, the mechanisms are very similar, but everything is in one piece. The cannula is still inserted under the skin with a needle, but there is no long tubing to connect pump to inset. The inserter, the cannula, and the insulin cartridge are all together, and the whole thing sits on the skin. It's larger on the body than the tubed pump inset, but again, there's no tubing, and you don't need to tuck it into a pouch or pocket. It does have an external controller you need to carry. Tubed pumps are operated by buttons or a touchscreen on the pump itself.

An insulin pump certainly isn't a cure, nor does it make diabetes management automatic. I remember feeling overwhelmed – would it be like learning diabetes all over again? From my blog, just before we started pump training in 2007:

I'm curious about so many aspects of this. How will he wear it? Most adults I know wear their pumps like a pager, clipped onto a belt or waistband. I've seen little kids with a kind of fanny pack to hold it on. I can't imagine my very active 2-year-old will tolerate that, but maybe he will.

The infusion site looks sort of like a nicotine patch with a bump on it once it's in. Benny doesn't even like Band-Aids ("Off, Mommy!"), so we'll see how he takes to that. *(Update: He never once complained about wearing it or messed around with it. I was shocked.)*

I just feel like this would be easier if Benny could really comprehend the advantages of the pump. At

2 years old, I can't tell him "no more shots" because he'll still get what feels like one every three days as we change the infusion site. Our diabetes educator, Linnet, was very reassuring. She says there are plenty of little kids running around with these pumps, and it works out just fine. We think we've decided on which brand to use. There are six companies that make different models. *(Update: There's actually less choice now.)* We'll get to see it up close, touch it, press all the buttons, and figure out if it's really the one we want to go with. Our insurance only pays for a new pump once every four years, so it's a big decision we'll live with until Benny's 6 years old. Six? Now I'm thinking about my little guy going to kindergarten with a pump. That's a whole other set of worry!

The pump visit with our certified diabetes educator (CDE) went really well. I remember that's when I actually started getting excited about switching to a pump. Our CDE has two sons with T1D, one diagnosed as a toddler, the other as an older teen. She knows her stuff.

Benny picked up the one we ultimately decided on and somehow got it to make music. He loved that! Like all pumps, the Animas 2020 had beeping alarms for when something needed attention, but it also played Beethoven's "Für Elise" for some alerts. There was a way to change that, but I never figured it out. You needed a dongle and an engineering degree.

Once we selected a tubed pump, we needed to also select an infusion set. As I mentioned earlier, that's how the insulin gets under the skin. I couldn't believe we had to make another choice. Angled or straight? Steel? Cannula length? Tubing length? The easiest decision was to use an auto-inserter. I was not ready to hand-insert the cannula, which is funny because we were up to about eight shots a day. Benny probably wouldn't have cared.

I told our educator to decide for us. I believe my words were, "Give us the best set that's also idiot-proof." She steered us to a purple auto-inserter that looked like a child's stamper. Then we tried it out on Benny. I say we, but I made Slade do it. I was worried it would really hurt and wanted to be the good guy if it did. We started with a Cleo applicator. It was discontinued a short time later, so we changed to the Animas inset. Now we're on the Tandem Auto-soft.

Benny reacted just like he does to a shot – no big deal. He's such a tough little guy. I was so excited and relieved. We decided to leave the little patch on his body, to see if it bothered him at all or if it came off as he ran around or sweated. (It shouldn't). My 5-year-old daughter wanted to check it out, and she thought it was pretty cool. Other than that, we didn't point it out at all, and he did great – took a bath, slept fine, didn't seem to notice it at all. It was a bit frustrating that after that step, we then had to order everything and set up an appointment to learn the system. It was about another month before we actually started.

Now, years later, I can say that for us, insets have been the toughest part of pumping. This is more pessimistic than I like to be, but they all stink. I'm not alone in this thinking. It took me almost a decade to figure out, but they are the weak link of pumping. If you put too much insulin through, they stop working efficiently too soon. If you don't put enough insulin through, they stop working efficiently too soon. They can bend, they can get blocked or occluded, and sometimes they don't go in correctly or stick well. We have fewer issues these days, but I still think there isn't enough attention paid to this part of pumping.

A lot of parents and caregivers will put on a pump inset to experience what it's like, or to show the child that it doesn't really hurt or even to show solidarity or empathy. Our day care manager did it, and I know loads of parents who have as well. I never could. I'm embarrassed to admit this, but I was afraid that if it did hurt, even a little, I'd never be able to put one on Benny again. I still feel guilty about that, but I know myself. I'm glad I didn't.

Overall, for us, pumping is worth it, even with the occasional bad site. The most important thing is to educate yourself about how insets work and what type is right for your child. As I mentioned, there are different kinds. Often, people who are thinner need an angled inset. Don't settle if yours isn't working. There may be a better type or a better placement.

When we got the pump, the transition did not go as planned. With all my planning and worry, I can honestly say I never thought Benny would grab his brand-new pump and throw it across the room. I cringed when it landed on our kitchen floor. He wasn't angry. Maybe in his toddler brain, it was simply a chance to throw something new? He never did it again, and the pump was fine, unlike my heart that had stopped for a few seconds. From my blog in June 2007:

> That Sunday afternoon, we set up the pump. Your doctor gives you a whole bunch of numbers to program in – insulin to carb ratios, blood glucose target numbers, etc. We did that, set up the tubing, and filled the pump cartridge with saline. We'll use saline instead of insulin until next Monday when we go "live" and start using it all for real. We got the inset onto Benny (we're calling it his "button"), and unlike last time at the educator's office, he was not happy about it. After the initial outburst (OK, it was a total tantrum), he calmed down until bedtime. When I changed him into PJs, he noticed the "button" on his tush and told me to "off it." Again, once we held firm, he seemed to forget about it. As of this morning, we haven't actually hooked the tubing to the inset, so he's not actually pumping, not even the saline.

After a few days on saline, we went back to the diabetes center and had a training session with a few other families. We were ready for the real thing. Or so we thought. The first problem cropped up a few hours into our visit, after Benny had eaten a few snacks and we'd dosed him with the pump. His blood sugar kept climbing. Finally we looked at the site, and it turned out I hadn't correctly connected the tubing to his inset. I'd attached it but not all the way. Nice job, Mom! I learned to firmly push the tubing end until I heard a "click."

They sent us home, and we felt pretty good the rest of the day. Benny didn't mind letting us take the pump out of its pouch to press the buttons. But that first night, again, his blood sugar kept climbing, so something was wrong.

At midnight, we decided to change the site. We actually debated going back to shots – it was a pretty tough moment. I remember whispering with Slade in Benny's room, hovering over the crib and debating whether to give a shot or change the site or both. We decided on a site change, and even though it woke him up, we all got back to sleep somehow. We needed the rest because we were traveling the next day.

Oh, did I mention that? Yes, we decided to start on the pump just before going to New York, where my parents spend the summer.

Here was my thinking: As you start on the pump, you need to check blood sugar more than usual. For us that meant at least every two to three hours around the clock. I thought that, with my mom around, she could watch the kids during the day while I caught up on sleep. That seemed to make starting the pump "on the road" not such a bad idea.

I hear you laughing already. Hold on.

In another genius move, we timed this out for the same weekend my husband goes away every year to play golf with his best friend in Vermont. I knew that without Slade, I'd be the only one who could take care of Benny and the new pump, but I wasn't really worried. We'd packed everything we needed. I could handle this. And I did. For about two days.

Along with changing the pump inset every three days, you change out – or really, replace – the insulin inside the pump. To replace the insulin with that model pump, you first remove the empty cartridge, having used up all the insulin inside. Then you use a special cartridge/needle combination to pull new insulin from a vial. That new cartridge goes into the pump, and after a brief loading and priming process, you're good to go.

It helps to bring a new cartridge. Apparently, we did not.

I checked everywhere. No cartridge. No special needle. That meant no way to put more insulin into the pump. That meant no more pump. I won't tell you who packed all the diabetes supplies, but his name rhymes with *played*, as in *played golf in Vermont* while I was freaking out in New York! Honestly, even with Slade away, I knew we'd be safe; we could switch back to shots. But first, I wanted to try everything I could to keep Benny pumping. We had just started!!

I called everyone: Slade, of course; our endo; Animas; and Linnet, our diabetes educator. The endo on call got back to us first and said we'd need a luer lock needle in order to get insulin out of the vial and into the old cartridge. My dad was on it. Out the door in a flash, I later learned he went to every pharmacy in the area. He wound up at a hospital! And they gave him the needle! I carried that stupid luer lock needle in my backup bag for years. My poor dad. But he is effective and resourceful.

Our educator, Linnet, came to the rescue. I love our endo practice, but it takes another diabetes parent sometimes to really get into the nitty gritty. Linnet politely acknowledged the luer lock needle suggestion was a good and proper one. Then she told me not to worry about it and walked me through reusing what we had on hand – totally off the books and not at all FDA approved.

Basically, we just reused the old cartridge. This pump compresses the cartridge to extract the insulin, so I stuck my fingernail into the ridge where it was pushed in on itself and was able to pull it back open so that we could put more insulin inside it again. No need for the special needle; we used a syringe I'd brought for backup to transfer insulin out of the vial and into the old cartridge. It took a while, and we had to wait until the air bubbles were out, but it worked!

Here's the wild part. The next day, Animas called my mom's house to tell her the New York rep was on her way over with the missing cartridges! No questions asked, no charge, just coming by to drop off exactly what we needed for the rest of our vacation and beyond. I was blown away by the customer service from these folks. I'd heard it was great, but who drives stuff to your house? Sigh. Sad to say, Animas is no longer in business; they announced their closing in 2017.

Meanwhile, Slade had actually found a family in Vermont with kids on the same pump! Again, remember that this was before social media. He and his friend had spent an hour calling friends and friends of friends until they found someone with T1D who used the same cartridges. He was ready to drive them to New York. Luckily, he didn't need to.

I can't say I'm happy we made that mistake, but forgetting those cartridges gave me new confidence. It was far from the last time we'd forget something or hit a snag with the pump or diabetes tech. Knowing we'd macgyvered our way through this situation so early on gave me confidence for the next mistake. It also solidified my trust in our doctors and educators. These are dedicated and special people. They were there for us even out of state and late at night. We were lucky to have such a great team.

The rest of the trip passed without any other major diabetes excitement. We swam a lot, and the kids went to the zoo and read books with their grandparents. The pump behaved, and the supplies were plentiful. We came home rested and ready to tackle the next diabetes mistake.

Knowing us, it wasn't far away.

ASK YOUR DOCTOR OR EDUCATOR

- Pump versus MDI – which one is right for my child? (Your endo and educator should help you make this decision, but ultimately, it's an individual choice. Don't feel pressured!)

- Do you have a paid relationship with a pump or CGM company? (This doesn't mean their recommendation is unethical, but it's good to know.)

- Can I see and hold each type of diabetes pump or CGM before I make a decision? (Learn about inset choices and tubing if you choose a tubed pump, and learn about the entire system, including the external controller, if you choose tubeless.)

- If my insurance denies my choice, do you have experience with appeals, and will you help me make that appeal?

- Do you have a packing list you'd recommend for travel?

CHAPTER 5

School Skills

As she talked about her fears, I felt my face getting warm. My heart pounded, and I squirmed in the little first-grade classroom seat. We knew this teacher – a wonderful, smart woman who'd challenged our daughter in the best way. I hadn't considered anything like this, especially since kindergarten had been smoother than I'd dared imagine. I wanted to jump up and yell. I could feel myself getting defensive and angry and readying a sarcastic comment.

By the time Benny started kindergarten, he'd been diagnosed with type 1 for almost four years. Even so, I was still very nervous about the transition. At the time, we knew he'd be the only kid with type 1 in the entire elementary school. Part of me was happy about that – I could teach them diabetes "our" way. But of course, that meant no one else really understood.

I did a ton of research, starting with our 504 plan. This plan refers to section 504 of the federal Rehabilitation Act of 1973. It's there to make sure any child with a disability at a public school receives accommodations that will provide support and remove barriers. You may have also heard of an IEP (individualized education plan), which is a bit different. An IEP provides more individualized special education and often requires more documentation. These are very simplified explanations of rather complex documents, so please check with your school and your doctor to decide what your child needs.

In our district, we also have something called a diabetes care plan (DCP). This lays out pretty much everything about how the child manages T1D; it's signed by your doctor and contains a lot of information that might be in other children's 504 plans. I mention it here because our experience with the 504 plan was really only for testing. We'd have a formal meeting each fall with Benny's counselor, the nurse, and lead or homeroom teacher. That meeting focused on end-of-grade and formal testing, which started in third grade for us. I considered it a bit of a warm-up as it helped us figure out what accommodations he did and didn't need by the time he got to middle school.

Of course, I didn't realize this in kindergarten, and I presented his school with a 10-page 504 plan with every accommodation I could think of! Ultimately, I'm glad I was over prepared. We were lucky with staff who knew our rights and were supportive and helpful. But having more documentation was reassuring to this nervous parent. I explained to the wonderful staff that they were wonderful, but I had no guarantee the next teacher or principal would be as wonderful. File the paperwork.

I wanted to meet with the school staff weeks before classes started. I knew they had already assigned Benny's teacher. We'd gone to a kindergarten orientation in the spring, and with Lea already at this school, we were acquainted with everyone there. Instead of weeks ahead though, we got Benny's teacher assignment and set up a meeting only about 10 days before school started.

I was slightly nervous. But boy were we lucky.

Miss Y had taught students with T1D before and was receptive to our way of doing things. Each kindergarten class in our school had an assistant, so she had an extra set of hands to help when needed. Under North Carolina state law, Benny was able to do all blood glucose checks and insulin dosing in the classroom.

His teacher even asked *all* parents not to bring in sweets or treats to celebrate birthdays. This wasn't about diabetes or specifically for Benny; she did it every year. She explained that kids have enough going on in kindergarten and that she'd appreciate it if a parent could donate a book and come in and read on the child's birthday. How great is that?!

The year wasn't without issues and setbacks. Benny found out breakfast was served at school. He didn't realize it was for children who needed the free meal. He just followed his friend in one day and got some cereal. This went on for about two or three days until the nurse checked in. She was worried about his unusually high midmorning BG check. Busted.

I felt so bad for Benny. Truly, he thought he'd committed a crime. There were some tears, and he was embarrassed and worried about what he'd done. We explained he just needed to make sure an adult knew if he was going to have an additional meal, so he could dose and be safe. And truly, he'd just eaten breakfast at home! He didn't need the free meal the school provided.

Overall, kindergarten was a time of learning and growing and managing diabetes in new ways. We had a few scary lows, especially as we got used to the timing of gym class and lunch, but nothing the staff couldn't handle.

We hit our first real school roadblock at the start of first grade.

At our back-to-school meeting, Benny's teacher admitted she was very nervous about his diabetes. Mrs. H. told us she wasn't sure she wanted him in her class. This was a big surprise; our daughter had been her student previously, and Mrs. H. had already agreed to teach Benny.

What happened?

Turns out, Mrs. H. had a relative in law school who wondered whether the teacher might be held responsible if anything went wrong. They'd had a few troubling conversations over the summer. The big worry: Would we sue if her diabetes management wasn't perfect?

As she talked about her fears, I felt my face getting warm. My heart pounded, and I squirmed in the little first-grade classroom seat. We knew this teacher – a wonderful, smart woman who'd challenged our daughter in the best way. I hadn't considered anything like this, especially since kindergarten had been smoother than I'd dared imagine. I wanted to jump up and yell. I could feel myself getting defensive and angry and readying a sarcastic comment. Thankfully, I stayed calm as Slade and I looked at each other and shifted into educator mode.

We explained the basics of type 1 diabetes. We talked about Good Samaritan laws and looked up the American Diabetes Association Safe at School Guidelines for our state. We pulled up North Carolina law and the school district policy. Luckily, I had done all of this research before kindergarten, so I knew where to find what we needed.

After seeing all of this information, Mrs. H. did a complete turnaround and became one of our biggest advocates. She welcomed Benny into her class and pushed the school to provide more help. The following year, our school went from one child with type 1 to four. The classroom assistant Mrs. H. pushed for became a floater who helped all the T1D kids manage.

I've learned that when someone throws up a roadblock, there is almost always a way around it. That way usually involves staying calm and educating. Is it tiring? Sure. Sometimes I feel like a broken record, but when I look back, I realize I'm not just advocating for my own child but also for all people with diabetes in the school district.

One of the ways we continued to advocate in school is by talking about diabetes every year to Benny's class. I started this when he was in preschool, and we did it every year until third grade. After that, it became less of an educational talk by me and more of a JDRF walk kick-off from Benny. I was relieved of my duties in this matter in sixth grade.

I wrote about my presentation when Benny was 6 years old and in first grade:

We started by reading Benny's favorite book about diabetes, "Jackie's Got Game." It's all about a boy with type 1 who wears a pump and checks his blood sugar at home, at school, wherever. He wants to make the basketball team, but would a low during tryouts keep him off the squad?!

For us, the very best part of this book is the final team roster. The first name on it is Benny! Unbelievable. Spoiler alert: Jackie makes the team.

After the book, I went a little further explaining what diabetes is and why Benny needs insulin. I kept it pretty simple for the kids: "Who knows how your body and brain get their energy, so you can move and think? Who here likes to eat food?"

Then Benny spoke and knocked me out. "Diabetes is awesome," he told his friends. "It makes me special."

I had never told him that. I do not think diabetes is awesome. However, hearing my 6-year-old be positive and excited about something that really could drag him down was about as awesome as it gets.

He checked his blood sugar in front of the class, just in case they hadn't seen him do it. He showed off his pump and picked two friends to touch it while I used the remote to bolus him, so they could feel it vibrate. ("I feel it!" they shouted.)

Then we opened it up for questions.

"Does Benny ever have a low number like the boy in the book?"

Yes. When he does, we give him juice or something with sugar in it to help get that number back up. He might not feel very well during that time, so please try to be a good friend and understand Benny might not want to play right at that moment. If Benny ever seems extra sleepy or slow, ask him if he feels OK and tell a grown-up. Thanks!

"Where do they get the insulin that goes into Benny's pump?"
Great question! Doctors make it in a special laboratory, and we get it at the pharmacy, the same place your parents get your medicine. Keeping it simple.
"Can Benny eat Cinnamon Toast Crunch?"
This is a very specific question. But yes, I measure it on a special food scale, so I know how much insulin he needs.

We chatted for almost 30 minutes, and then it was time to go. When I got home Slade was just back from the grocery store. With cereal. I kid you not. He'd purchased Cinnamon Toast Crunch – 22 carbs an ounce!

Another challenge we faced at school was food. I packed lunch and included the carb count for every item, along with a total. At a younger age, Benny would dose after lunch, with supervision from his classroom assistant or teacher. As he got older and we trusted he would really eat what he thought he'd eat, he'd dose before eating.

What he really wanted was to buy lunch. For whatever reason, buying the cafeteria lunch is very popular at our elementary school; Lea bought lunch at least three days a week. Of course Benny wanted in. We decided to make it happen and jumped into planning. Here's what we came up with (from my blog):

I will print the school menu with all the carb counts the night before. This is a pretty cool feature they've had for a few years now. (It also includes allergens). Benny and I will decide what he wants to eat and circle those items.

I'll provide a list of "backup items" in case they run out of the strawberry-applesauce he wants, and he has to eat grapes or carrots.

His class assistant will walk him through the line to see what goes on his tray, and she'll check in with him after lunch to see what's left over, just like she does now. If she's not available, one of the cafeteria workers has volunteered to help us out.

Just like now, the assistant will do the math, and Benny will use his pump to give himself the insulin.

We did a test run and found that roughly a quarter of items on the food line weren't listed on the district carb menu. I looked those items up on my own and provided the counts. I also found out that fruit servings are always 4 ounces (helpful) and that most of the desserts are only about 15 carbs (not too bad). Our school district has done away with fried foods and provides lots of whole grains, fruits, and vegetables.

Of course, Benny is only excited about eating what I think are the worst foods on the menu: corn dogs and nachos. I can't pretend we eat perfectly healthy at home all the time, but these are never served in my house, which is probably why he wants them! However, I'm willing to trade off some high-fat high-carb lunches – and probably some higher afternoon BGs – for a pretty important step toward independence.

Eventually, he'll have to make his own food choices, count his own carbs, do the math and give his own insulin unsupervised. I don't think first grade is too early to start working on that. I am extremely lucky to have such a great team helping me with Benny.

At first, he only bought lunch once a week. By fourth grade he was much better at carb counting and dosing, so we let him buy whenever he wanted. By middle school, he was back to only wanting packed lunches. Fine by me! Easier on the carb counting and less guesswork. But then we knew he could pretty much eat anything and make good dosing guesses.

Every state has its own policy about dosing and checking at school. As I mentioned, the American Diabetes Association (ADA) Safe at School website is a terrific resource to find out what the rules are where you live. In North Carolina, kids are allowed to carry all of their diabetes supplies, check BG, and dose wherever they are in school. They don't have to see the nurse for everything.

We trained a few staff members and teachers on glucagon and showed them how to supervise Benny on checking and dosing. Our part-time nurse was excellent and reassured other staff that they could do this. In fourth grade we hit the jackpot with a nurse who lives with type 1.

We didn't get the Dexcom Share phone app until fifth grade, and at that point, we decided there was no need to share with the nurse or other staff. That's a tough decision, in my opinion. I've heard from parents who love it and find school staff to be receptive and appropriately responsible. I've also heard from parents who find staff to overreact and pull kids from class at every beep or alarm. And some districts are becoming more cautious about letting staff follow BG information from any personal devices. It's worth a few conversations before you jump in and invite anyone else to look at your child's diabetes data.

One thing that really helped us in those early years was that Benny was definitely a rule follower. He hated anything different or special and didn't want to miss out on activities or class time because of diabetes. But sometimes, that made things a bit more difficult. From my blog in 2014 when Benny was in third grade:

> The morning forecast said flurries by noon, maybe an inch of snow. I live in the South, so we knew that meant school would be getting out early. I put a PowerAde and a protein bar in a brown paper lunch bag.

"This is your emergency snow-day snack-pack, dude." I reminded Benny that early dismissal means coming home on the bus, just as usual. I wasn't anticipating trouble – we live less than fifteen minutes from the school. But I wanted him to know he had supplies in case traffic was crazy or the bus was late.

"So if you go low on the bus, you have lots of carbs here. Drink the PowerAde first."

"But Mom," he said, "can you call school and tell them? Because you're not supposed to eat on the bus."

Sigh.

"We've talked about this. With diabetes, you eat when you need to. The bus driver knows. Remember just last week when you were running late? You'd already bolused for breakfast, but you hadn't finished, and you took your cereal in a bag onto the bus? And it was fine?"

"Yeah, but could you write it down, so everyone knows?"

That's when we sat down and talked about the 504 plan and how it's written down for everyone to see at school. How I'll always have his back, so he shouldn't worry about standing up and speaking out if he needs help. How he can tell the bus driver to call me or even yell, "Medical emergency!" if he needs to.

We also talked about suspending the pump if he's low, or even disconnecting altogether. He's never had to do that at school or on the bus, but I like to know he knows his options. I reminded him that he always carries juice or Quick Sticks glucose in his meter pouch (duh, Mom).

We've had this talk several times since kindergarten, and I expect to keep talking about it until he's an adult. How he feels and acts at 9 is not the same as how he was at 6 or how he'll be at 12. These conversations need to continue and change with his age. Of course, I haven't changed a bit. Right?

Benny has always taken the bus and – knock on wood – we haven't had any issues. He likes to follow the rules, he doesn't want to get in trouble, and he doesn't want to use diabetes as an excuse. This drives me a little crazy. Who cares what the bus driver thinks? Just drink the damn juice box if you need it! But it mostly makes me very proud of my son who doesn't want special treatment.

As predicted, the snow fell, and schools dismissed early. The bus pulled up and snow-crazy Southern kids poured off. The snow-day snack-pack went back in the cabinet, untouched, ready for next time.

Something else that's helped, especially as Benny gets older, is a quick talk at the beginning of the school year about what he really wants. Beginning in middle school, he didn't want to check in with the nurse or any faculty about dosing and BG checks. He was allowed to carry his cell phone to use Dexcom Share during the day, which helped.

We set parameters. I'll text if his blood sugar is above or below a certain number for a certain amount of time. If there's an urgent low alert, which means BG is 55 or under, he has 15 minutes to text or call – or have someone else text or call – before I start blowing up his phone.

I text him every day, 20 minutes before lunch, with a bolus reminder. I'm surprised that he still wants this since he goes to high school this fall. But when I asked him about it, he said, "Mom, I have enough to worry about at school. If you can take care of the lunchtime diabetes stuff, I can take care of school stuff."

I wanted to point out that he's still taking care of the diabetes stuff – I'm just sending a reminder. But if it works for him, that's great for me.

I highly recommend at least a yearly talk with your child

about their goals and needs each school year. Younger children love to feel like big kids with more responsibility, and you may be surprised what they share about their goals and thoughts about T1D.

Older children just want to know we're listening to them, that we take their wants seriously and that their opinions matter to us. Benny rolls his eyes at me during some of these talks and jokes around, but that's just teen brain. I know he appreciates that he has a say.

ASK YOUR DOCTOR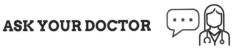

- What are the laws and policies about type 1 diabetes in my state and local school district?

- What paperwork does my school district require?

- What school care plan do you recommend? (Ultimately, this should be a decision reached as a team by parents and doctors.)

- Do you have any recommendations for changing dosing because of my child's school schedule, such as when gym or lunch fall?

CHAPTER 6

Caregivers

When Benny changed the cartridge, he followed my directions very well, including the part where I wrote in capital letters REMOVE THE PUMP FROM YOUR BODY BEFORE PRIMING THE PUMP. He did that. But he didn't actually *detach* the pump from his body by removing the tubing from the inset. He just took it out of the little pouch around his waist and put the pump on the kitchen counter. That's *removing it from the body*, right?

"Which parent is home to watch your son during the day?" the doctor asked while looking down at his clipboard.

"Neither one of us," I snarled. Then I burst into tears. After a long day of rushing to the hospital, watching my kiddo go through pokes and tests and rip off the sensors like a baby hulk, this was the question that put me over the edge.

I was in my dream job, hosting a top-rated morning radio news show in a terrific city. I'd busted my butt doing TV news in small towns, working long and lousy hours, and I finally had a job that was fun and rewarding and high profile. It was a dream. And I saw it going away.

How could I work? We'd always had help. I loved our day care, the socialization, the fun, the caring people. And what about health insurance? My husband owned his own business, a restaurant, so I was the steady earner and the health insurance provider. What were we going to do?

As I cried and the horrified doctor wondered what the heck he said to set me off, Benny reached over and patted me on the shoulder. "It'll be OK, Mommy," he said softly. Hoo boy. When your not-yet-2-year-old is trying to make YOU feel better, it's time to get a grip.

I wiped my eyes and sat up straight. I gave him a big hug and pulled him onto my lap. "I'm sorry," I told the doctor. "I'm just not sure what we're going to do; we both work."

"Well, he has type 1. Lots of kids with type 1 have day care or nannies," said the doctor. "You'll work it out." He smiled at me, relieved he had some reassurance for me. And he was right.

For most of my career, I worked very early mornings. First in local TV news, then at a radio station. Every city has one – we give you the news, weather, and traffic every 10 minutes on the 10s. That meant I left the house around 3:30 a.m. every morning. I did that for 13 years.

My husband was almost always home in the morning. Since he owned a restaurant, his afternoons and evenings were a mess, and we traded off. However, sometimes he traveled, and I would have a neighbor or a friend stay overnight, so I could go to work. I even had one sitter who would come over at 3:30 a.m. if needed!

My wonderful neighbor Jackie helped us like that just before Benny turned 7. He was in first grade. Jackie has two adult children with type 1, which is how we met, but they were diagnosed in their early 20s, and she doesn't have a lot of hands-on diabetes experience. She does have a huge heart and is a smart cookie; she's the kind of child caregiver you dream about, diabetes or not.

As we were getting ready for bed, we realized Benny would need a pump cartridge refill. He had more than enough to make it through the night but would run out sometime after breakfast. I started to change it out, just to make it easier on everyone, but

Benny stopped me. He wanted to do it himself. "Miss Jackie will be there if I need anything!" he argued.

Benny knew how to change a cartridge but had never done it without me or Slade around. I wrote out step-by-step instructions that night and left for work in the dark as usual.

I was hosting the show myself that day; we were doing the show in a coffee shop where I'd meet listeners while my producer was back in the studio. I was also at least an hour away from our house. Knowing all this, Jackie didn't text me until about halfway through this episode – when (spoiler alert!) everything was fine.

Here's what happened. Benny woke up and changed the cartridge, and then Jackie helped get both kids ready for school. She drove them, and just before they got to school, Benny said he didn't feel very well. She parked and walked them in, sending Lea to her classroom. Benny sat down in the hallway and didn't want to move. Of course, she checked his blood sugar. He was low, around 70. They treated with the usual 15 carb juice box, waited, and checked again. He had gone lower, down to 50.

Jackie alerted the school nurse and took Benny to the school cafeteria. They hung out and ate for about an hour until his BG started to come back up.

So what happened? You've probably guessed.

When you change out the cartridge in a tubed insulin pump, there are several steps. You remove the pump from your body by unclipping the tubing from the inset. Then you fill the cartridge, check for air bubbles, go through a few steps so the pump recognizes and acknowledges the cartridge, and then prime the pump, which usually involves sending some insulin through the tubing and confirming that it drips out of the end. Then you reconnect the pump tubing to the inset on the body.

When Benny changed the cartridge, he followed my directions very well, including the part where I wrote in capital letters REMOVE THE PUMP FROM YOUR BODY BEFORE PRIMING THE PUMP. Benny did that. But he didn't actually *detach* the pump from his body by removing the tubing from the inset. He just took it out of the little pouch around his waist and put the pump on the kitchen counter. That's *removing it from the body,* right?

No. It is not.

Since the tubing was still attached, when he primed the pump, all of that insulin went into his body. The Animas pump we used at the time took at least 12 units to prime. Keep in mind, this is a first-grader who maybe weighed 50 pounds. For perspective, at that time he probably didn't dose more than a unit or two at most for anything he ate or for a BG correction.

I had a choice. I could have dropped everything and run home – I'm not sure what that would've sounded like on the radio, but they would've made it work. My job wasn't in danger. I knew, though, that there wasn't anything for me to do. The danger had passed, his blood sugar was beginning to go up, and he was already talking about going to class by the time Jackie clued me in. He stayed in school the rest of the day. By the time I saw him, everything was back to normal.

If eating everything in sight hadn't worked, or if Benny hadn't felt well enough to eat or drink, this would have been a good time to use a glucagon emergency kit. Glucagon is a hormone that helps your liver release its stores of glucose, which raises blood sugar. The glucagon emergency kit contains a powder form of the hormone and a syringe filled with liquid. You mix the two together and inject. That's a very simple explanation of a complex and important diabetes tool. It also requires a prescription, so please ask your doctor more about when and how to use it.

We were lucky that Benny enjoyed his snacking excursion in the cafeteria and that his blood sugar didn't sky rocket for the rest of the day. But poor Jackie felt horribly guilty. Years later, she still talks about it, but I can never be upset with her. She took care of him. She stayed with him. Something went wrong, and they dealt with it.

A word on babysitters while we're here. Like a lot of people, we were happy with the neighborhood teens when the kids were little, but that changed for us after diabetes. I felt that 2 years old was too young to leave him with someone not familiar with T1D.

It's a tough call. An articulate 5-year-old who can check his own BG can be fine for an evening with a "regular" sitter. A newly diagnosed 11-year-old may need more help. In general, I like to say all you really need is someone who cares and pays attention, but there are a few things you can do to make it easier.

We'd give the kids dinner before going out if possible, so we could dose and minimize the BG checks. Or we'd portion out snacks and count carbs ahead of time. I wrote up "action plans" to help with the process. They were mostly simplified "if this blood glucose, then that action" type of directions.

I should mention that I did pay my sitters more after than before the diagnosis. We went from 14-year-olds to college students and adults. Our day care providers were a great source for sitting – two were even nursing students! They also had the advantage of seeing Benny every single day, so they were more used to the T1D routine, even if they weren't in his classroom or helping manage diabetes every day.

As I mentioned in Chapter 3, we were lucky that our day care center was friendly about taking Benny back after his diagnosis. I joked with Rebecca, the manager, "Do you think he could sleep here?" because they already had a girl with type 1 at the center, and it seemed like Rebecca knew more than I did!

While we were in the hospital, I was very worried about our child care. Slade and I both worked full time, and our children had been in the same place for a long time. They had friends, and we all loved the staff.

We met with them and looked at the other child's guidebook, and I realized I needn't have worried so much. About a week after we came home from the hospital, we sent Benny back to day care. At the time, the manager was the only one who could do shots and check BG, and we set up a schedule. They made hot meals at this center, so we did the best we could figuring out carb counts and dosing. We had a kit we brought back and forth, and they'd write all the dosing and BG checks on his daily care sheet that went home with every kid. They worked with us; we worked with them.

Other options are finding siblings of T1D kids, T1D teens or using a service like Safe Sitting, which specializes in connecting T1D-savvy sitters to families. We found one of our best sitters – who's now a dear friend – through a regular babysitting/nanny service. I called them up and asked if they had anyone comfortable with T1D, and they had a couple of young women who were!

Many of my evenings out were for work – I had events that I was expected to attend as a "local personality." It was tough with Slade working nights but an important part of my career. We did try for the occasional fun date night or just an afternoon away together. And it's important to acknowledge that the costs of all those babysitters can add up. But date night is really important, as is time for yourself. I've seen communities have luck with a babysitting co-op, where parents trade time. They don't have to be all T1D families either. Again, that's up to you. If your child can count carbs, check BG, and dose insulin with supervision, you can probably teach a sitter everything they need to know.

We always invited a new sitter over for dinner first, so they could watch Benny in action and learn about diabetes. Usually a meal is a good illustration of the ins and outs of diabetes.

We also found sitters were much more receptive to helping out after we switched to an insulin pump. Maybe that shouldn't have surprised me, but it did. After all, a pump is a complicated bit of machinery, and using it incorrectly can be dangerous, as we found out! But most people prefer to press a button than to stick a syringe in a little kid.

Everyone hated giving Benny shots. A few people apologetically refused to do it. It's not why we got the pump, but once we had it, we realized it made people much more comfortable. The same people who asked not to give shots, were happy to press a button. Benny didn't care if you gave him a shot as long as you didn't ask him to stop playing; he would just pick up his arm, wouldn't even look at you. But his caregivers loved not having those needles.

Along the way, we also made our own luck. Our JDRF chapter offers caregiver training once a year. This is usually a daylong session geared toward grandparents, babysitters, coaches, and teachers – anyone who helps care for a kid with type 1. It might be sponsored by a pump company or underwritten by fundraising. But anytime we heard about one of these, we sent any potential sitter who might be interested. We paid them, but honestly it wasn't a lot. They truly seemed to want to learn.

I remember asking a potential sitter to check out the caregiver training when Benny was about 3 years old. When she told me she was excited to go, I burst into tears. We were in front of a whole bunch of people, and I just started tearing up. Everyone wanted to know what was wrong. Turns out everything was very right. From my blog that day:

> It's hard to describe how much it means that people are willing to learn about diabetes to help care for my kids. I'm sure it will get easier as Benny gets older and can use his own pump and check his own blood sugar. But right now, he needs more than a sitter. He needs a helper. And how lucky are we that so many want to be that for him.

We did have one more bit of cartridge excitement about two years later. Benny texted to say that he was going to refill his cartridge while we were out. We had one of our regular, knowledgeable sitters. Thankfully, Benny removed the pump completely this time. But then he filled the pump with Lantus – a long-acting insulin that he was NOT supposed to use in the pump. We keep a bottle of long-acting in the fridge as a backup in case there are pump issues. He'd grabbed it by accident.

We were already on our way home, so we caught that one before he'd even bolused a drop. After that, I separated the backup insulin to avoid any confusion. That would've been a tough 24 hours until the Lantus was out of his body, but we would have dealt with it. Almost everyone I know has mixed up long- and short-acting vials at least once. Here's a quick tip I got from a CDE I spoke to on the podcast. Wrap a rubber band around the pen or vial of long-acting insulin and leave the short-acting pen or vial unwrapped. After a few weeks, your hands should instinctively feel the difference before your mind knows which type you've picked up.

Lea is three years older than Benny, so after she was old enough, we felt comfortable leaving them home alone together. That was also just about the time Benny started wearing a CGM and when the Dexcom Share app came along. That's a game changer when it comes to parental comfort.

With any game changer, though, there are ups and downs. Using a CGM that allows you to remote monitor helps us troubleshoot and respond to high and low alerts. But we find it can also tie us more to home and make it hard to go out and disconnect, which is why you have a babysitter in the first place.

ASK YOUR DOCTOR

■ How do I know if my child is ready to check BG on their own or start working toward more independence and responsibility?

■ What are the best ways for us to treat severe lows?

■ When and how should we use a glucagon kit?

■ Are there accommodations or care changes you would recommend when a sitter is in charge, such as adjusting our blood glucose target range?

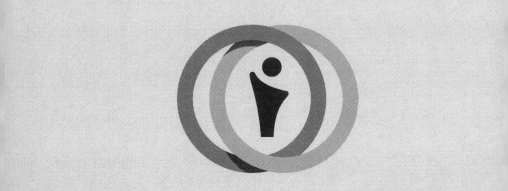

CHAPTER 7

The Backup Plan

"The pump says there's only one unit left,"
Slade said. What? How is that possible? Why
didn't the pump alarm go off? Oh, wait … that's
when I remembered Benny waking up at 1 a.m.,
stumbling into my room muttering, "My pump's
making noise." The reminder alarm was going off,
indicating the pump only had 10 units of insulin
left. I confirmed the alarm, which turns it off, and
told him we'd change the cartridge in the morning.
Of course, in the morning all I remembered was
that I was pretty tired for some reason.

How many restaurants have we walked into and *beep, beep, beep* the no-insulin/empty-cartridge alarm goes off? Or an inset comes out at the pool, and you don't want to leave just then? While I never like that feeling of "fix it later," we've learned that Benny is more resilient, and diabetes is less of an emergency than I ever thought it would be during those first few scary months after diagnosis.

My husband likes to say the backup plan is more important than the actual plan. That came in handy when he was a TV newscast director, which is how we met. We've found it to be very true for diabetes in action.

One day, in fourth grade, Benny called me from school. "Mom, my inset came out." I was planning to leave work just a few minutes later, but I was still at least a half hour away. My husband was at a doctor's appointment, and I knew we wouldn't reach him for a while. Besides, Benny didn't really need our immediate help.

"Go ahead and change it yourself," I said, shutting off my computer and grabbing my car keys. "I'll see you after school." He said OK and hung up. But a few minutes later my phone buzzed again. "There aren't any insets in my backup bag."

Really?

I asked about blood glucose. It was on the higher side but still in range. He felt fine, so I told him I'd be there soon and to go back to class. We had a part-time nurse for most of Benny's elementary school years, and she wasn't there that day. But the school staff is wonderful. I knew he'd be fine until I could get to school.

I keep backup diabetes supplies in my car, so I didn't have to stop at home to get what I needed. I don't have everything for every situation, but I keep at least an inset or two, along with glucose tabs and snacks in a plastic pencil case. I almost always have Gatorade or a juice box, some bottled water, and a few other bags of nuts or granola bars stored somewhere as well. I like a well-stocked car; my husband jokes we could survive for a week on what's in it!

I drove right to school, and we changed the inset and, as it turned out, didn't have to bolus. He'd been playing pretty hard at recess, and the Dexcom arrow was pointing down.

I checked the school backup bag, and it was a mess. As Benny said, it had no more insets and was low on test strips, and if I had to guess, I'd say the lancer in the backup meter kit hadn't been changed since the first day of school. I took this as a sign that Benny had been using the supplies (which is great!) but not telling me (which is not so great). After putting a reminder in my phone to actually bring the bag back to school the next day, we headed home.

With situations like this, we have a choice. I could've written a stern email to the nurse about making sure the supplies are stocked. But in my opinion, that's our responsibility. I could have had Benny sit in the front office until I arrived and whisked him out of school, regardless of where his BG was. And I could have yelled at him for not paying more attention to everything.

But mistakes and problems can be good lessons. Benny learns that he can handle bumps in the road, with support. Soon enough, he'll be on his own, and he needs to know that most difficult situations with diabetes will not be disasters. It's also good for his teacher, who still gets a little nervous when numbers get wonky or diabetes doesn't behave. It's also great for the office staff. They know that it's important to keep us posted and informed, but they've learned they can handle a lot of situations better than they might have thought. Of course, there's so much more that goes into good diabetes management, but it starts with caring about the child and simply paying attention.

We repacked the bag and sent it back to school. I put another reminder in my phone to check with the nurse monthly to go over supplies. I've got new insets in my pencil case in the car. We're ready for the next time something goes wrong.

Another time, we needed backup when we took the kids snow tubing. Slade and I grew up in New York, but our children are snow-deprived. The Charlotte, North Carolina, area gets maybe 1 to 2 inches a year and rarely all at once. We're more likely to get ice or slushy yuck. Once every couple of years, we get 3 to 4 inches all at once, and the kids go bananas.

That day, we bundled everyone up and headed off to the mountains. I packed two changes of clothes and extra socks and shoes for everyone. We don't have actual winter clothes (no ski jackets or pants), and I assumed there'd be a lot of slush and wet. I also threw in our diabetes bag.

Benny carries his meter and a juice box wherever he goes. For most of elementary school, he used a leather pouch. It's really a golf tee/supply bag, but it's a great fit, and Benny doesn't feel like he's carrying a purse. When we take a day trip or will be out for a while, I throw a bigger diabetes bag in the car. It's a dopp-kit that can hold our pump supplies, extra strips, insulin, needles, and so forth. In the summer, I put the insulin vial in a Frio, a handy little pouch that uses the cooling power of evaporation to keep the insulin at room temperature. Somehow, it all fits.

A day outside in the mountains meant stopping on the road for a big breakfast. Our kids love the Waffle House, and I've resigned myself to eating there. (I try not to watch the grease on the grill.) After ordering something smothered and covered, Slade and Benny figured out the carbs, and Benny started to bolus. They both looked up at me with that "something's wrong" look.

"The pump says there's only one unit left," Slade said. What? How is that possible? Why didn't the pump alarm go off? Oh, wait … that's when I remembered Benny waking up at 1 a.m., stumbling into my room muttering, "My pump's making noise." The reminder alarm was going off, indicating the pump only had 10 units of insulin left. I confirmed the alarm, which turns it off, and told him we'd change the cartridge in the morning. Of course, in the morning all I remembered was that I was pretty tired for some reason.

I walked to the car with my heart in my throat. I had the diabetes bag, so I knew we should be all set. But while I was reassuring Benny everything would be fine, I was trying to remember if I'd double-checked the bag and if I could even remember the last time I'd reloaded everything. We were at least an hour from home, and I have to admit that I was nervous. But it was all there. One quick cartridge change in the car and a giant breakfast bolus, and then we were on our way to tubing.

I'm not sure what I would have done if we had no insulin. Maybe gone home. Maybe chanced it for the day, hoping all the activity would keep BG in range. We definitely would have changed his Waffle House order.

I supposed I could have called around to nearby pharmacies. We use a national chain, so it's possible they could have filled a prescription. My fear there would have been whether our insurance would cover an extra vial.

Now, with social media, I probably could have found someone in the area with an insulin pen. But back then, it would never have occurred to me to try. These are the situations that make diabetes so frustrating. You don't want it to stop you, but being without needed supplies (really I'm talking about insulin here) can create a dangerous situation. Remember that he was pumping and only using short-acting insulin at this time, so there was no long-acting basal in his body. I'm comfortable with a lot, but a full day away from home without insulin would probably have been over my limit.

What should you keep in your bag? How big of a bag do you need? As usual with diabetes, it depends.

Many kids wear a little sling bag. In fact, when I see that small sling bag from Amazon (some of you are nodding), I always give a second look to see if I can spot a pump or CGM. That's actually how I recognized a friend at our local amusement park. Her kid ran by me, and I spotted "the bag." Then I saw her. The kids were mortified, but we thought it was great. Hi, Tiffany!

When Benny was little, we carried everything back and forth to day care each day in that dopp-kit. We left a few backup supplies there, but it was easier to have everything we needed wherever Benny was.

In elementary school we switched to having him carry that pouch with low-sugar supplies and his meter. The nurse kept all his diabetes gear in her office and insulin in the fridge. His classrooms had juice and snacks put aside just for him. The go-bag still went with us everywhere.

In middle school, Benny started carrying a small backpack when he went out without us. This is when we switched to putting an insulin pen in the bag. I would write the no-good date on the pen (28 days after taking it out of the fridge) and make sure there were some pen needles in his pack. Then if he needed insulin in his pump, he could take it from the pen or inject.

(Note: Once you suck the insulin out of the pen with the pump cartridge needle, you can no longer use the pen to inject. Air can get in and mess with the dosing.)

Here's what's in Benny's bag right now:

- Meter case with meter, strips, alcohol pads, lancer, and lancets
- Low-sugar treatment such as glucose tabs, gummies, and/or honey packets
- Glucagon emergency kit
- Insulin pen and pen needles
- Portable charger and multicharger cable that works on both his pump and his iPhone
- Two pump insets
- Two pump cartridges

It's probably more than we need, but it's handy when he calls after hanging out with friends and asks if he can stay the night. It helps us say yes if he's got everything he needs.

I go through Benny's bag about once a week to make sure the supplies are actually there and the insulin still good. As he gets older, he'll take on more of that responsibility, but it helps me let go if I know he has what he needs.

There will be a next time, of course. And that's why the backup plan is just as important as the plan itself.

ASK YOUR DOCTOR

- What's a good backup plan if we forget something?

- How do you recommend we carry insulin? Pens or vials with syringes?

- What should be in our "backup bag?"

- Is the insulin prescription written to allow for an emergency or "vacation" refill? (You may have to ask your pharmacist about this as well.)

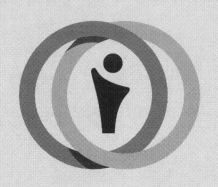

CHAPTER 8

Numbers and Nerves

I've come across a lot of people in the diabetes community who are natural math people. They keep great logs and are fluent in numbers. I'm good at math. I took AP calculus in high school, I balance my checkbook, and I can time a 60-second commercial break without a stop watch. But diabetes math has always tripped me up. That's because when you need more, sometimes it seems like you need less.

I think diabetes likes to lull us into a false sense of security. Just when we start to think we know what we're doing – BAM! Something knocks us over.

About a year into Benny's diagnosis, we were checking Benny's blood glucose several times a day, sometimes as many as 8 to 10 times during the day and overnight. Very standard operations: We used a lancer to prick his finger and get a drop of blood. That goes onto a test strip inserted in a meter, which gives us his BG number.

The test strips come in little cylindrical containers. They look almost like mini versions of what 35 mm film used to come in.

Do you shake yours? I shake the container each time before I open it. I have no idea why. I find that little sound somehow reassuring.

Each little container has a "code" number on it. When you put the test strip into the meter, the same number should come up. On our meter you have to manually reset that number each time you change containers. After that, you can just press "OK" on the meter when the number comes up. We'd been doing this for about 10 months (wow), and we knew the drill. Or so we thought.

For about two and half days we were getting unusual and erratic BG numbers – 95 one hour, then 405 an hour later when Benny hadn't eaten anything, or 250 overnight and 350 in the morning. It just didn't make sense. We didn't know if the pump was broken or if Benny was going through some kind of toddler growth spurt or even getting sick. Finally, Slade figured it out.

Seems that when I changed from the #11 canister to the #17 canister, I mixed up the numbers and never reset the meter – 17 looks just like 11, right? We got lucky. The only time Benny really got low was right after Slade figured out the problem and checked him. After a quick juice box, we were off and running.

Matching the codes – or finding the right codes and setting for your meter – is obviously important. No meter is 100 percent accurate, but we want them as close as possible. Even though we now use a continuous glucose monitor (CGM), it's still vital to have a backup or another way to check BG. I joke around a lot about being the worst and making mistakes, but the more I know, the more this episode scared me. We could have easily over treated for those false high blood sugars.

We had another mistake, but kind of a silly one, one night later. We would usually check Benny just before we got to bed, when he'd been asleep for a while. I'd go into his room, juggle a small flashlight, prick his finger, and get the number. We would treat or dose accordingly. Believe it or not, he usually slept through it. That time, though, it took me five test strips. Of course, it woke him up, and he was sleepily telling me to give him the flashlight. When I did, he turned it off! This was one of the late-night BG checks that led me to buy a headlamp – yes, a headlamp like a coal miner. At least when I got his BG, I knew the number was accurate, and he was even in range.

Several years later, I got another reminder that I'm not quite the diabetes expert I like to think I am. At that point, we'd been using an insulin pump for almost eight years. We had a terrific endo visit that month. Labs were normal, A1C was low, elementary school life was fine, and Dr. V talked to Benny about baseball season coming up. But about a week after we walked out of the office, it seemed like all of a sudden Benny's BG shot up and stayed high.

I sent Dr. V three weeks of Dexcom reports, and he recommended we adjust the insulin sensitivity factor (ISF) overnight. We hadn't looked at the ISF in a while, so that made sense. Dr. V said, "Go ahead and make it stronger," so I did. Or so I thought.

The ISF is also called the correction factor. It's the amount blood glucose is lowered by dosing 1 unit of short-acting insulin. You need it to figure out the amount of insulin to give when your blood sugar is high – it's the equation you use to get back down into your target range. An example – and how it looked in the pump we used at the time – is "1U:50." That means it takes one unit of insulin to bring your blood sugar down 50 points.

I've come cross a lot of people in the diabetes community who are natural math people. They keep great logs and are fluent in numbers. I'm good at math. I took AP calculus in high school, I balance my checkbook, and I can time a 60-second commercial break without a stop watch. But diabetes math has always tripped me up. That's because when you need more, sometimes it seems like you need less.

Case in point is this ISF. If you need to make it "stronger" as my doctor suggested, you need to lower the second number. But in my brain, less doesn't mean more. MORE means more. You always keep the 1U part the same, so if he needed more insulin, *of course* you'd change the second number to a bigger number. Right? Nope.

I initially changed the correction factor to 1U:60. But when you break it down, that mean he's getting less insulin. We needed to change it to 1U:40, and after a little confusion, I realized my mistake.

I feel foolish admitting it, but I know I'm not the only one. In fact, when I Googled "insulin sensitivity factor," it took me several tries to find an explanation that was easy to understand. It doesn't help that it has two names. Our educator confirms this is very common.

I do the same thing with insulin to carb ratios. It's hard for me to grasp the concept that smaller numbers mean more insulin. I'm not going to say I'm bad at math, but this is a concept that I have to concentrate on to get right. It's like saying the D in Wednesday every time I spell it. You do that too?

For great explanations of all of this, and so much more, I highly recommend the book "Think Like a Pancreas" by Certified Diabetes Educator Gary Scheiner. He breaks these concepts down so that they're easy to understand and gives you some terrific charts and resources to use. He also updates the book every few years to include the latest in technology.

We fixed the correction factor and ultimately wound up increasing the basal rate as well. If you did the math on Benny's age, you might realize that he was just about to enter puberty. That's a different story and an altogether different book! In fact, there's already another book I'd highly recommend called "Raising Teens with Diabetes: A Survival Guide for Parents" by Moira McCarthy.

A few weeks after all of that adjusting, we spent a school holiday away. Benny's Dexcom sensor was hanging by a thread when we started the trip. I knew it would be coming out while we were away. Normally, this wouldn't be a big deal, but Slade didn't come with us on our trip. Since we started using the Dexcom about a year and a half prior, the only people who'd inserted the sensor were Slade, Benny, and a counselor at diabetes camp. I'd never done it.

Slade does a great job. He's fast, like all the advice says you need to be, and he and Benny have a routine. It's to the point that if Slade's got a late meeting and the Dexcom comes off, we'll just wait until the morning. It's a little weird since Slade and I have been a pretty 50-50 diabetes management team for all this time.

So while I brought sensors with us, I didn't expect Benny to let me put one on. And that would've been OK. I love using the CGM, but we'd managed diabetes for seven years without it. So while a couple of days without it would've felt odd, we would have been fine.

To my surprise, Benny said he was ready for me to give it a try. "I'll set it up, Mom," he said, helpfully pulling the tape off the inserter and positioning it on his stomach. "You just push the plunger, pull it out, and be fast. Like Dad." He removed the "safety" and looked at me expectantly.

I love Dexcom. Let me say that. Using a CGM can be life changing, and we were one of the very first families to receive and use the G6 system – the newest system as of this writing. It has an easy insertion that requires just one hand and a quick button push. It's accurate and works with our insulin pump. Having said that, the G5 and previous Dexcom inserters were terrifying.

If you've used one or even seen them, you know what I mean. The inserter is gigantic and awkward to use. It's not natural to insert the way you're guided. You have a plunger and a collar. You're supposed to put your fingers above the collar for insertion and then switch and put your fingers below the collar to pull the plunger back up. The instructions even say, "Insertion will not feel natural the first few times."

First few times? I only had this one time to get it right! I willed myself to be calm. "No problem, dude," I said. "Let's do this."

He pinched up his skin (which helps) and counted three … two … one. I pushed the plunger, but as I pulled back, he said, "Mom, you're done! Stop! You're going to yank the whole thing off." I was working so quickly, I had already pulled the plunger back without realizing it.

"That was great, really fast! You were even better than Dad," Benny said as he clicked off the applicator and popped the transmitter into the new sensor.

"I have to tell you something," I said. "I was really nervous."

"Then you should always be nervous, because that didn't hurt one bit. I can't wait to tell Dad!"

It was nice to be back on the team.

ASK YOUR DOCTOR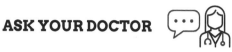

- Does our meter need to be coded or calibrated? If so, will you show me how?

- Can you write out any changes you've made to pump settings or injection dosing? Why have those changes been made?

- What BG results should I look for in the next few days or weeks once these dosing changes have been made?

- Do you recommend any online instructions or how-to videos for CGM or pump site insertion?

CHAPTER 9

On-the-Road Adventures

Lea was in tears. "I want to get wanded!" Did she think this was a magic wand? What was going through her 5-year-old brain? I looked back at the TSA lady, finished with Benny and about to start with me, then back at my teary-eyed daughter. She didn't really know what was going on, but she knew she was being left out of something because of diabetes. Using the poor judgment only a frazzled parent can show, I gestured to Lea for her to come quickly. She jumped down, ran over, and hugged me. The TSA lady turned around, and for one moment, I thought maybe we were all going to TSA jail.

Our first big trip with diabetes was uneventful. Just three weeks after Benny was diagnosed, we got on a plane. We already had the tickets, we had the time off, and we went. Traveling with little kids is a circus already, so we decided that diabetes was just another flying trapeze act to add to the show.

We are very fortunate to be able to travel several times a year, and we've even traveled internationally. We'll pick up and drive long distances and once RVed from North Carolina to Chicago, cruising through six states in five days. We've found a lot of things that work for us, and of course, we have had quite a few bumps in the road.

Let's pack up, and I'll tell you what we've learned.

Driving

Driving usually means lots of sitting still. If you change your activity level, you likely will need to change your insulin dosing. We've found that if the trip is over two hours, we need to give more. It's much easier to do this with an insulin pump.

If you've done this using your insulin pump (every make and model of pump has this option even if they call it something different), you know how easy it is. But if you've never done it before, it sounds like a lot of math. At least it did to me.

I held off for a long time on using the advanced features of Benny's insulin pump. We only had the one day of pump training, and everything seemed good enough to us. Then I attended a conference where the speaker talked about using temporary basal rates on insulin pumps, specifically for travel or for illness.

Lucky for me, I was seated next to our certified diabetes educator (CDE), Linnet, who was also attending the conference. I asked her what she thought; would a temporary basal rate be a good idea for a long car ride? She said it would and scribbled some notes, including trying a 25 percent increase. At that time, Benny had about five or six different basal rates, not uncommon for growing kids.

I sheepishly admitted that I wasn't sure how to do all the math, asking if I just multiplied all the separate basal rates by 0.25. She looked at me like I had three heads. Then she laughed.

"Stacey, the pump will do that for you!" She explained. "You just tell it 25 percent more or less and for how long, and it's done!"

Oh. That sounded much easier. We tried it and never looked back. We use temporary basals for all sorts of activity now – or lack of activity. It can make for a good math lesson if you want your child to really think things through, but it's as simple as she said. Just make sure you talk to your endo or CDE about finding out what's right for you.

I was very conservative at first, raising the basal rate 15 percent and checking every 20 minutes. Now, when we drive eight to 10 hours at a time (not uncommon for us), Benny cranks it up to 80 percent or even more sometimes. We usually start two hours before the trip and end about two hours before we arrive. Of course, your timing may vary.

Long car trips with a child in a car seat do make using an insulin pump a bit more difficult. Before we started using the meter remote, it was a bit of a contortionist act. This was back when Benny was strapped into a car seat and too young to use his pump by himself. "Don't crash," I'd tell my husband before I moved the passenger seat *way* back. I'd flip my seatbelt off, turn around, and grab Benny's pump for a quick bolus. I definitely do not recommend this, but if I'm being honest, it was the easiest way to keep things moving.

Snacks on the road are tough with or without diabetes. We pack a cooler with the kids' high-protein, low-carb favorites, but those just aren't as much fun as gas station junk food. So we do indulge a bit. On that drive to Florida, we usually stop once for snacks, once for a real meal and once *just for gum* – enough already!

It's a good idea to keep diabetes supplies within reach. You don't want to be zipping down the highway, finally making good time, and realize you need something in the trunk. While most kids have their own diabetes bag, I usually pack an additional small bag with a day or two of supplies and throw it in the front seat with us. We use it while we're driving and also as a just-in-case bag. We've been stuck in some nasty traffic jams, and I don't want to be without insulin or an extra cartridge for hours at a time.

We also bring a football or a Frisbee, so we can get out of the car and run around every couple of hours. We've done jumping jacks, run laps, anything to just move for a few minutes.

Flying

The worst airport experience we've had so far was one of our first with an insulin pump. We had just wrapped up a vacation with extended family in Vermont. Benny was 2 and had been using his pump for about two months. Lea was 5.

TSA asked us to empty the entire diaper bag. Not poke around and look inside it. Take everything out. I piled up diaper cream, diabetes supplies, sippy cups, wipes, and probably 20 loose toys and Legos and books.

Then they wanted to wand Benny. My husband was well behind us, having been stopped for his own TSA inspection. He has a prosthetic knee, so we were used to leaving him behind for a bit at airports. In fact, knowing his dad got special treatment at the airport made it easier to explain to Benny why he now needed extra attention too. I agreed to let them wand Benny, but of course, he wanted me to hold him. He was 2 and didn't really have any idea what was going on.

The TSA woman didn't want me to touch him. "If anyone touches someone in this zone – she indicated a small circle on the floor – then they have to get wanded." She made "wanded" sound like the worst sort of punishment, as though instead of just having a TSA staffer pass what's basically a stick over your body, someone was instead going to dump a bucket of burning sludge on you. I told her I'd do my best. But as I tried to sort of hold Benny up without actually holding him, of course he jumped up and wrapped himself around me.

The TSA lady was not pleased. I told her I had no problem getting wanded, and we would just take our time. Then I looked over to check on Lea. She was in tears. "I want to get wanded!" she cried. Did she think this was a magic wand? What was going through her 5-year-old brain?

I looked back at the TSA lady, finished with Benny and about to start with me, then back at my teary-eyed daughter. She didn't really know what was going on, but she knew she was being left out of something because of diabetes. We were less than a year in, but Lea had already realized that her brother experienced a lot – good and bad – that she could not.

Using the poor judgment only a frazzled parent can show, I gestured to Lea for her to come quickly. She jumped down, ran over, and hugged me. The TSA lady turned around, and for one moment, I thought maybe we were all going to TSA jail.

"I'm so sorry," I said, gesturing to the little circle of doom on the floor. "I know she has to be wanded now. We'll wait."

I think she was just happy to get rid of us. She wanded me, then Lea, and then we moved on. Slade had rejoined us at that point. Thankfully, even though he had no idea what was going on, he just helped me repack everything, and we all got to the gate where I explained. It sounded just as ridiculous then as it does now.

Besides not aggravating the TSA people, there are a few things you can do to make your experience a bit easier.

Be early! You already know that, but it really makes a difference. This is especially important if you wear a pump and/or continuous glucose monitor. It's hard to predict how quickly you'll get through security. We've had trips with no issues whatsoever, and we've also lost 30 minutes when the TSA worker didn't know what an insulin pump was and had to call for her manager.

Find out the policy for your diabetes technology, or "d-tech" as many people call it. Get in touch with the company that makes your pump or CGM and print out the airport security policy. The safest policy is to request a hand inspection. Most metal detectors are fine, but your tech may set it off, making a hand inspection necessary anyway. And most cannot go through the full body scanners many airports now use.

Expect inconsistencies. We've had everything from a brief wanding to a full patdown. Once or twice they've asked Benny to handle his pump, and then they wipe down his hands and test that. We've learned that hand lotion or even soap residue can set things off. One time they wanded and checked his shoe laces!

Each time I say, "Wow, every time there's something different." And the TSA agent always says, "Nope, it's pretty consistent." Sure it is.

We used to carry ice packs and try to refrigerate the insulin everywhere we went. That's still helpful if your child is on very small amounts. But insulin can stay potent at room temperature for 28 days. Now we travel with a Frio cooling wallet, which keeps the insulin cool but not cold, and an extra pen or two. Whatever we don't use on our trip, we're able to use back home. TSA policy is to allow ice packs if they are fully frozen, but not if they are melted and mushy. Again, check before you travel.

If you do have a young child with diabetes, explain a few days before what might happen. I'd go so far as to pretend to pat down or wand your child. Since my husband (with the metal knee) has always been taken aside, my kids knew the drill before diabetes entered the picture. If they didn't, though, it could be little frightening. Explain you'll be there every step of the way and that the airport helpers are just there to make everyone safe.

We paid for TSA Precheck a few years back, and I feel that if you travel more than once a year, this is a fantastic service, definitely worth the cost of $80 for five years. There is no charge for children under 13 if they travel with someone who has Precheck. If you want more personalized help, call TSA Cares. That's a helpline that provides travelers with disabilities, medical conditions and other special circumstances additional assistance during the security screening process. We have never used it, but on their website, they say you can "call 72 hours prior to traveling with questions about screening policies, procedures, and what to expect at the security checkpoint." The number is (855) 787-2227.

Bring much more than you think you'll need and keep it with you. Project Blue November has great packing lists available through their Facebook page. We carry our diabetes supplies in a bag that doesn't leave my sight. I usually throw one or two days' worth of extra supplies in my daughter's or husband's carry-on, just in case.

Most airlines allow you to have a small medical bag in addition to the carry-ons they allow. It's worth looking into. You may even want to print out the policy – not every staffer is familiar with every rule and regulation. It can be frustrating but is easier if you're prepared.

Of course, expect the unexpected. We once sat on the tarmac for 6.5 hours before a 1.5-hour flight. This was before Benny was diagnosed with diabetes; he was a little over a year old, and my daughter was almost 4. Yes, it was a nightmare.

My husband made hand puppets out of the air sickness bags to entertain Lea. We read every book in our bag to the kids, and we colored, and we were miserable. This was before smart phones and before we traveled with any sort of movie player. Benny was terrific and barely fussed during that whole ordeal. But once we got in the car, he screamed his lungs out all the way home. Good timing, kid!

That nightmare flight has stayed with me. I think about it every time I pack, and it's one of the reasons we stopped flying for a while. Diabetes can make travel a bit more challenging, and our days of packing light are most certainly behind us. But being prepared makes all the difference.

How ever you travel, be careful of the hour or so just after you get off the plane or out of the car, train or bus. Walking around, playing hard or jumping into your hotel's pool can really get the blood pumping. The increased circulation moves the insulin around and makes it work much more efficiently than it has been for the past few hours while you've been sitting still. If you've stacked a lot of insulin doses or even given some large boluses in just the last hours of your trip, you might be in for a crash.

We had a trip home once where everyone except Benny slept through the meals on the way back. He ate his meal, his dessert, and probably half the snacks on the plane. "I bolused for everything, Mom," he told me proudly while I struggled to wake up and return my seat to the upright position.

Even with the dosing, he was 400 when we walked off the plane and headed to our connecting flight home. Twenty minutes later, when we had walked to our faraway gate, his BG was 45. Insulin likes circulation.

You may also want to disconnect your pump for takeoff and landing. Some research suggests that many insulin pumps are affected by pressure changes during takeoff and landing, which can result in unintended dosing. The amount of insulin here is small – maybe a unit more or less – but that is a lot for children and any adult who's very sensitive to it.

Like most people, we got a note from our doctor indicating that Benny has diabetes and that we needed the syringes, insulin, and other gear we were traveling with. I kept that note with us for 10 years. No one ever asked to see it. But I wouldn't advise against carrying it. When it comes to travel, I'd rather be overprepared.

ASK YOUR DOCTOR

- Whether MDI or pumping, should I change any settings for specific travel?

- How do I set temporary basal rates (if using an insulin pump) and when should they be used?

- What supplies do I need for travel?

- Do you have a suggested diabetes supply packing list?

- Do I need a doctor's note for travel and can you help me make a list of prescription information I may need if out of town?

CHAPTER 10

Brothers and Sisters

It was our first moment of realizing how much diabetes was going to push us to give Benny more attention. Lea had been looking forward to ice skating for weeks. Here in the South, that's an exotic activity and something she'd never actually done. But Benny had just been admitted the night before. We hadn't yet met with his endocrinologist. What kind of mother leaves her not-yet-2-year-old son in the hospital, even if his father is there, to go ice skating of all things? *Sigh*. This kind.

When I shared our diagnosis story earlier, I left out one important part. While I was preoccupied with worry and learning and planning for our new life with type 1, my mind was also on ice skating.

Earlier that year, we had helped form a brand-new temple in our area. In fact, until Benny's diagnosis, Slade and I thought that was where all of our extra attention outside of work and family was going to go. I had planned a fun holiday outing for our members at an ice-skating rink in Charlotte just a few minutes from the hospital but about a half an hour from our home. That outing was set to happen our second day in the hospital.

I knew everyone would understand if I didn't go. However, the rink was operated by my radio station as a holiday promotion; I was the only link between the two groups. Since I had arranged it all, skipping would be confusing and complicated. More importantly, Lea really wanted to go.

It was our first moment of realizing how much diabetes was going to push us to give Benny more attention. How would we handle the balancing act of a child with a chronic condition with making sure our other child didn't feel left out at every turn?

We talked it out. Benny was acting fine and seemed to be feeling better than he had in ages. Twenty-four hours on insulin will do that! Lea had been looking forward to ice skating for weeks. Here in the South, that's an exotic activity and something she'd never actually done. But Benny had just been admitted the night before. We hadn't yet met with his endocrinologist. What kind of mother leaves her not-yet-2-year-old son in the hospital, even if his father is there, to go ice skating of all things?

Sigh. This kind.

Even as I felt the guilt of leaving Benny, I knew it was the right decision. All these years later, I remember what that cold fresh air felt like as we walked out of the hospital. I grabbed Lea's hand and smiled at her.

Trying to give your children equal attention is a bit of a losing battle, even without a chronic illness. But once something like diabetes comes into the picture, there are simply times when one child needs more attention than the other. I remember putting both kids to bed and – if Benny's blood sugar was low or he needed a pump inset change or whatever – just giving Lea a book and telling her I'd be back in soon. I always felt so guilty about that, but Slade just wasn't home most nights, so it had to be that way. I'm sure he had similar moments in the morning.

Lea stepped up pretty quickly, like many siblings of T1D children do. She would run to get the meter or tell me when she thought Benny didn't look right. It was sort of like when her little brother was born. She'd get me a diaper or sit with him on her lap for a few minutes and sing to him. Then she'd get bored or frustrated because he didn't want to "play" with her. Totally normal big sister behavior.

She and Benny also started playing "hospital" a few days after we got home. Lea wasn't the doctor; she was the patient in those early days. There was always a mysterious illness that required an overnight stay but never a shot. The stuffed animals were always the ones who needed to get a bolus or a blood sugar check. From my blog in 2007:

> As we all got more comfortable with diabetes, it was easier to include Lea a bit more. She was fascinated by checking blood sugar and drawing up insulin. She was not happy when I wouldn't let her give her brother the actual shot, though. And she's very good at letting us know if Benny eats something when we're not looking! I know it's important to reinforce the idea that our family is a team in dealing with this.
>
> We've always monitored our kids' diets pretty closely. I never kept chips or juice around, but we did have occasional treats and desserts. Now, though, we've gone from eating almost whatever we want, whenever we want, to measuring and counting every single thing Benny eats. Since we count carbs for Benny, for a while we were even afraid to give him fruit. We've come to our senses, thank goodness. How can you teach a 2-year-old that an apple or a banana is a treat to be restricted along with chocolate or sweets? Benny has decided that cantaloupe is his favorite right now. I'm trying to get him to call it "lope." He calls it "soup." But, see, even here when I started out talking about Lea, I came right back to Benny. And that's what worries me.
>
> I think we have to acknowledge and accept that he will get more of our attention, but also convey to

her that she has our undivided support and, of course, our unconditional love.

That sisterly support was tested when Benny started kindergarten and took the bus to school. The kids are three years apart in age but, because of where their birthdays fall on the calendar, four years apart in school. Lea was in fourth grade and, year by year, had been making her way to the back of the bus where the cool, older kids sit. When Benny went to kindergarten, the driver asked him to sit right up front, directly behind the driver. Then he made Lea sit next to Benny!

The seat assignment didn't come from us. We had talked to both kids about looking out for each other, explaining that's what brothers and sisters do, not only with diabetes but also in all aspects of life. Of course, that includes the school bus. But the driver wanted to make extra sure Benny was safe, so he did what he thought was right and easy – make his sister sit with him.

After a week or two, she finally told us. At that point the driver was a bit more comfortable, and we reassured him that Benny's friends would all look after him. They wanted to sit with him too. So Lea got to move back with the other "big" fourth graders. It might sound silly but was very important to her at the time.

We tried to make sure that we each had one-on-one time with Lea. I would take her for an annual overnight, just us girls. Or we'd go to dinner together. Slade would spend time with just her going to the movies or doing projects around the house. When she was older, they found they really enjoyed cooking together.

I think what really helped with Lea is that we never tried to make excuses or pretend everything was "normal." Sometimes diabetes just demands priority, and that stinks all around. It's OK to tell your other child that. My parenting style is about honest communication. That includes saying, "I'm sorry I can't do that with you right now." And then listening when she wants to complain about it. I want to complain about it too!

Making time for her alone or even just deciding that Slade would be in charge of diabetes if we were all together at a school event, so I could give her my full attention, went a long way in showing Lea that we were there for her too. Just saying these things out loud is important. You may think your children just know, but they may not.

In 2016, after 10 years of diabetes, I interviewed Lea for my podcast about her experience as a sibling of a child with T1D. She was 15 at the time and shared that she definitely remembered feeling upset that Benny got so much more attention.

"It's not that I didn't understand what it was, but I still wanted more attention," She told me. "He needed you guys, and I knew diabetes was awful, but I wanted more. Pay attention to meeeee!" she laughed. She told me she was happy we'd talked things out with her a lot. It was helpful to know that we understood and acknowledged that things didn't seem "equal."

Interestingly, she never remembers being scared by diabetes except once. When she was just a bit older, maybe 10 or 11, and I showed her the emergency glucagon kit. "You want me to stab my brother?!" she remembers thinking. I remember her being incredibly calm and seeming responsible beyond her age.

Overall, during that interview and since, Lea has said that while she still doesn't think all the extra attention Benny got was "fair," she understands it and has long since made her peace with it.

There was one time at least that diabetes paid off for Lea. In the spring of 2013, Nick Jonas filmed a movie not too far from our home. Nick, of course, is part of the Jonas Brothers, who got their start on the Disney channel and are huge on the pop-rock scene. He was diagnosed with type 1 diabetes at age 13.

Nick agreed to do a meet and greet with some local kids. Lea and Benny were invited, and it was a *huge* deal. For Lea. Benny was not impressed. At age 7 his response was, "Nick Jonas is for girls." Of course, we went anyway.

It turned out to be a crazy day. We had to wait outside because the amusement park where they were shooting wasn't yet open and no buildings were unlocked. It started to rain, and everyone got drenched. The park and PR people brought us towels and brought around cars to take us to the set. The pictures are very funny – a bunch of smiling, wet kids with yellow towels standing around a completely dry Nick Jonas.

It was very brief, but he was very gracious and spoke to everyone. Lea asked him about the movie; he said he wasn't sure she would be allowed to see it because he thought it might be PG-13. She asked me to look into that and showed me Nick had signed her cell phone case. Benny asked when Nick was diagnosed, and they chatted about their respective ages then and now. Then it was over and time for him and the crew to go back to work. That was six years ago, and Benny has never let Lea forget how much diabetes helped her out that day!

I was hardly thinking positive thoughts about diabetes back during that first weekend in 2006. But when Lea and I stepped out of the hospital together and made our way to the skating rink, it just felt right.

I can't describe how much our friends' hugs, smiles, tears, and support meant. No one knew exactly what we were going through or what Benny's diagnosis meant. Neither did we at that point. Of course I was worried about Benny. Of course I cried a few times on the ice. But skating around with my 5-year-old, falling a couple of times, and then drinking hot chocolate was a much-needed reminder of all the good stuff.

What a gift that time was. That two hours of fun and skating with Lea set the tone for years to come. Diabetes was in our lives, but she knew we wouldn't let it take over. She knew she wasn't going to be left behind.

ASK YOUR DOCTOR

- Are there any local programs for children who have a sibling with type 1 diabetes or another chronic condition?

- Are there any diabetes camps in our area that encourage siblings to attend?

- Do you recommend my other child(ren) take part in any diabetes care? If so, what aspects would you recommend based on age?

CHAPTER 11

The Beach

Benny tried to reconnect his pump and realized
he couldn't. The tubing end just wouldn't go back
into the inset. We couldn't get it to click into place.
Slade took a look and realized the inset was full of
sand. I immediately knew what happened – and felt
my heart sink because I also immediately knew I
could have prevented it.

We take a family vacation to the beach at least once a year.
Sand and surf mean taking some care with Benny's
insulin pump, but we got used to that pretty quickly. In fact, by
2010 when this episode took place, I thought we had beach time
under control. Oops. Diabetes is just full of surprises.

We packed up the kids and the car and headed back to our
favorite place, Isle of Palms, South Carolina, affectionately known
to many as IOP. We hit the beach before we even unpacked – the
kids splashing in the waves, a family walk on the sand, digging
holes and building castles. Exactly what we go there for. I felt my
blood pressure go down just watching the ocean meet the shore.

At this time, we were using the Animas insulin pump, which
was waterproof, but we almost always took it off while swimming
and always in the ocean. When he was younger, Benny's blood
sugar usually went low during swimming, and ocean water is

not recommended for any insulin pump as far as I know. So we'd disconnect on the beach and reconnect every now and then.

Ask your health care provider to teach you the best way to do this for you or your child. You want to make sure you don't miss out on too much basal insulin. Our endo recommends checking BG and reconnecting the pump at least every two hours.

That night, we headed to dinner straight from the beach. We didn't even change, just threw some dry cover-ups over our suits; IOP is that kind of place. We always go to Luke 'n Ollie's, a fun, casual place. My husband has known the owner since their days at summer camp together in New York. We ordered and then took out all the diabetes stuff to dose.

Benny tried to reconnect his pump and realized he couldn't. The tubing end just wouldn't go back into the inset. We couldn't get it to click into place. Slade took a look and realized the inset was full of sand. I immediately knew what happened – and felt my heart sink because I also immediately knew I could have prevented it. All tubed pumps come with this little piece that you click in when you disconnect the tubing for bathing or swimming. I used it once or twice but didn't see the point; we never had any trouble before, and I knew I'd just lose the tiny clip-in. Now – at the beach, with a suit full of sand – I got it. Of course, we didn't bring any little click-in thingies with us.

With dinner already ordered, we talked about alternatives to simply changing the inset. We had all our supplies with us, but Benny was very reluctant at that age about any extra shots or inset changes. Could we dump water in it and rinse the sand out? We poured a bottle of water on it, but that didn't wash enough sand out. Years later, we did have success with that – what, you think this is only time we forgot? – but that was in the shower, not something we had access to in the restaurant.

We ended up changing Benny's inset before dinner arrived, but then had the issue of knowing we were just at the start of our beach vacation with no thingies. (I believe they are called pump clips, if you want to get technical.) I was stumped, but Slade came up with a great idea. Since the clip is basically the same thing that's at the end of pump tubing, why not just use that? We change the tubing every three days, and I'd brought extras. He cut off the tubing from the old inset we'd just changed, leaving a few inches dangling from the end. He tied a knot and ta-dah! New pump clip.

It wasn't pretty. Benny had a little bit of extra tubing and a little knot sticking up like a bump, but my kids wore rash shirts at that age, so it was covered up. Besides, Benny didn't really care as long as he knew he could play on the beach and jump through waves.

Side note: I didn't stop at the time to think about what the other people in the restaurant must have thought. We were at an outside table, jumping around, pouring water down our son's bathing suit. Just another day in the life of a T1D family!

Couple of thoughts here: First, if that had happened today, we would simply have given Benny a shot and moved on. One of the worst things I did (for real) out of ignorance was stop doing shots entirely when we switched to a pump. I would highly advise you keep insulin shots – pen or syringe – in your repertoire. Otherwise, you may find your child, like mine, forgets that they weren't really bothered by shots and becomes terrified of them.

Insulin shots are much better at treating a high blood sugar than waiting around and wondering if the pump inset is working or not. They are great if a pump stops working altogether or if a pump cartridge runs out of insulin. Benny started doing his own "backup shots" around age 10 when he wanted to take a pump break. I told him he had to do shots because I wasn't following him around all day to do them. It must have been the right time for him because he took a deep breath, steeled himself, and gave himself an insulin shot. After that, it was much easier.

If you switch to a pump, consider giving a shot of fast-acting every couple of days instead of a pump bolus, just to stay familiar with them. Ask your doctor about correcting by shot when your child is over 300 and/or when you're not sure about the pump inset. Older children may not need this "shot upkeep," but when you're diagnosed as a toddler, you don't remember a lot about those first few months. Many little kids who tolerated shots with no issues at age 2 or 3 become terrified of them by age 7 or 8. It can be like starting all over again.

Now that Benny is comfortable with shots again, we throw an insulin pen into his backup bag. If he runs out of insulin in his pump, or there's a question about the inset, he can decide to take a shot.

He can also, and this will make some people cringe as it's not FDA approved, pull the insulin out of the pen to use in a pump cartridge. Once you do that, though, you can't use the pen for shots. Pulling the insulin out results in air being pulled into the pen, which can affect dosing. I also always write the "no-good" date on the pen with a Sharpie, and when it gets close to 28 days, we make sure to use it.

By the way, isn't "28 Days Later" a zombie movie? I always picture zombie insulin marching around if I miss the date.

At the zombie-free beach, we like to bring a small hard-sided cooler with us. We always store our meter and other diabetes gear in something like that. You want to keep it cool, and of course, it's an easy way to bring along drinks and any other snacks for treating lows you may need. I usually put the d-tech in plastic bags inside the cooler to protect everything from condensation and sand. When we got a CGM, we kept this routine the same. CGM receivers, phones, and pumps don't work as well when they get too hot, and insulin itself can become less effective in extreme heat. It doesn't have to stay cold, but it can't get hot.

Getting diabetes gear to stick when you're at the beach or pool can be tough too. We have tried everything, and you may have to as well because everyone's skin is so different.

Overlay patches work well for some people. Several brands are available, many with fun shapes and designs. We found Stay Put brand is great for Benny's skin, as is the Dexcom branded overlay. We also find using skin prep liquid like Skin Tac works very well to keep things on day to day. Opsite Flexifix tape has always been our go to for insets – I just cut a little hole before sticking it on.

Many people find success with Vet Wrap or Sleek Sleeves brand if you wear the CGM or inset on your arm. (It's not always FDA approved, so check with your endo.) Benny never liked that, but I think it's a great option, especially Sleek Sleeves that can be used over and over again. You can order most of these items online through Amazon or in their own retail shops.

We find a plain old waterproof Band Aid works great, but they're tricky to remove without pulling off sites. We save that for days when we really need to protect the Dexcom sensor. Swimming in the incredibly salty Dead Sea is a good example. We covered the entire site with a Tegaderm clear bandage.

I've shared the knot-in-the-tubing trick quite a few times since then with families who also had no idea what those little pitchfork things are. For a while, I traveled with two pump clips in Benny's meter case, and after that trip, they were always in our swim bag.

But that first time, as usual, we figured it out. With a plan in place and insulin delivered, we enjoyed dinner and that great sleep I only seem to get at the beach. For the rest of our trip, we worried less about diabetes and spent more time teaching the kids to fly kites and boogie board. It was a great vacation.

P.S. If you're ever in IOP, check out Luke 'n Ollie's. Make sure to ask Jonathan about his big win on "The Price Is Right." You could also ask to see the office/closet where we changed Benny's site, but that's not on the menu.

- Can I get an additional prescription, or can you write our prescriptions for certain supplies so that we have backups for trips or even at home? Do you have samples of anything we use?

- Do we have a prescription for long-acting insulin as a backup for our insulin pump? Have you written a prescription for pen needles or syringes to go along with this pen or vial?

- If we disconnect our child's insulin pump at the beach, how often should we check BG and reattach the pump?

- Can you go through our diabetes supplies with me to make sure I understand what each item is and what it's for?

CHAPTER 12

Summer Camp

I woke up every morning at 4 a.m. in a cold sweat, convinced I had made the biggest mistake of my life and his life too. How could I have sent Benny away to "regular" camp? Didn't I know he had diabetes? Every bad scenario, big and small, ran through my brain. What if a low stopped him from having fun? Would the other kids make fun of him or exclude him? What if something really bad happened, and no one helped?

"**M**om, don't take this wrong, but sometimes I like camp better than home. I wish the future was here today, and I was already back."

Let's talk about camp. Not just diabetes camp, which is what 8-year-old Benny was talking about there, but all the camps. If you haven't thought about sending your kid to non-diabetes day camp or to a non-diabetes sleepaway camp, let me walk you through what worked for us.

Diabetes camp is a special place. Not only does almost everyone there have diabetes, but also it's often the first chance children with type 1 have to be away from their parents. Some have never spent more than a school day out of their mom's or dad's care. Studies show children with T1D who attend diabetes camp have better health outcomes later in life. Most adults I know with type 1 say it gave them a community before they could even realize why such a thing is important. In fact, they liked it so much or wanted to have another chance to attend that there are now several adult summer camp experiences.

Diabetes Programs

Let's talk about diabetes day camp first. We are fortunate enough to have two day-camp programs in our area, one each by the local endo groups. They're really just three-day weekend programs, but for many parents, it's the first time their child is in someone else's care. I started an annual breakfast event where the new parents could come and cry, and the experienced parents could start enjoying!

"Camp KUDOS is the best thing we do all summer," Benny told me when he was about 6 or 7. "Because there's nothing else where everybody has diabetes."

Here's what I wrote in my blog the summer that Benny was 4 years old:

> Many children at Camp KUDOS have never spent a full day away from their parents. Others, like Benny, don't spend much time, if any, with other children with diabetes. He loved it. His counselor, Josh, was a young guy, a Charlotte fire fighter with type 1. Benny just loved him. (What 4-year-old wouldn't?)
>
> I was excited because Benny now wears his medic-alert bracelet. Boy, has that been a struggle. I wish I'd slapped it on him when he was first diagnosed. He just has not liked the way it feels, or something. We just told him he couldn't go to camp without it. Done. And he hasn't taken it off since. However, this isn't really a rule at camp. We got into a little trouble when Benny told every kid he saw without a medical ID bracelet that they

weren't supposed to be there! Luckily, the counselors somehow sorted that one out.

The only snag came a few days after Camp KUDOS ended. Benny got very upset with us. He insisted camp was still going on without him. It took a while (and a lot of tears), but we finally convinced him that it was just three days and that we would never, ever let them have Camp KUDOS again without him.

A few years later, Benny was eager to try the local diabetes sleepaway camp. Our program is a week long, about an hour and a half away from home. The counselors at KUDOS had told him all about it, and it lived up to the hype:

> "At camp, there was a zip line, and your butt hit the water when you went over the lake!"
> That's our 7-year-old just home from one week at diabetes sleepaway camp. It was Benny's first extended time away from us. I wasn't concerned about his safety; this is an American Diabetes Association program with doctors, nurses, and trained staff. I was worried he'd miss home (and, OK, that I'd miss him).
> We dropped him off on Sunday. I held out until Tuesday. I know several people there, so I put out a couple of messages over Facebook and by text. Our diabetes educator made it clear Benny was having a great time, and I made it clear I wouldn't text again.
> "At camp, there was a giant banana slide and a big pool!"
> I had modest hopes for Benny's time at camp: make new friends, learn more about diabetes, and maybe change his own pump inset once. The staff works hard to meet the family's goals, but I had my doubts about that one. Wouldn't you know, they actually got him to try it.

The counselors talk about positive mental attitude (PMA) quite a bit. Benny got high marks for his and came home doing cheers and songs about it. He was also really proud of being the boy in his cabin who had diabetes the longest – five years. (Yay?)

"At camp, I was the loudest when we cheered at the rally. We won because of me." (I believe this. Dude had no voice when we picked him up!)

Now that Benny is home, he's looking at labels and asking about what's on his plate. We're pushing him to continue checking his own blood sugar and using the pump independently all the time. He's done this at school for the past two years (and even his last year in preschool), but we've let him lean on us at home.

He changed his own insulin cartridge today, and tonight we put in the new inset without numbing cream "because that's what I did at camp." If you've read this blog, you know the inset is one of our biggest challenges. It's hard to explain how much progress this is; I had to turn away because I had tears in my eyes.

Here's what else I love. Benny's favorite memories of this past week have nothing to do with diabetes. It's the zip line, the slide, the pool, and his new friends. Yes, of course he knows why he went to that camp. He knows he shoulders more responsibility than his "regular" 7-year-old friends at home. But now he knows there's a place where he doesn't have to think about being "different." Because at camp, he isn't.

Another terrific side effect of diabetes camp is seeing all the technology other kids use. Benny started on a pump at age 2 but wasn't really interested in a CGM. After two years at diabetes camp he decided to give it a try and brought it up at our late summer endo visit unprompted. He also saw other children wearing pump sites in different locations. When he was ready to test out using his leg, he FaceTimed a friend who walked him through it. These are experiences he couldn't get at home with me.

"Regular" Day Camp

The same year Benny started at diabetes sleepaway camp, we decided to send him to a local "regular" day camp. Up until then he'd been going to day camp at the day care center where the kids had gone since they were babies. Neither my husband nor I had the summer off, and we loved the day care program. But my daughter had started moving on around the same age, and we wanted Benny to have those experiences at well.

I started communicating with the camp in February of that year. While they hadn't had a child with type 1 in the day camp that they could remember, they did have a T1D kiddo in their after-school program. They agreed to work with us so that Benny could have a fun and safe experience.

Their counselors would not administer insulin, change insets or check BG. They would supervise Benny's actions in doing so, and since he couldn't do his own pump insets or shots at the time, we knew we'd probably have to go to camp once in a while to help. While there wasn't a nurse or medical staff on site, there were several people trained in basic emergency care.

I wrote up simple diabetes action sheets for Benny and his counselors to follow. We had a schedule of BG checks; the kids all brought lunch and snacks every day, so we knew what he'd be eating and could include carb counts. I also knew ahead of time if there was ice cream or pizza for a special day and included that information as well. I printed up the sheets, put them in laminated folders, and stuck them in Benny's lunchbox every day.

Those "action sheets" were also signed by our endocrinologist. We talked with him about camp and what he thought we needed to do. It was helpful to have his input, and having him sign off on these non-formal forms went a long way to making everyone feel better about the plan.

I think it's important to acknowledge that we were pretty lucky here in that the camp was only 15 minutes from my house and that my husband and I worked odd hours, which meant one of us could usually get to camp within the hour if something went wrong. We were also lucky that we found a staff willing to take on these extra responsibilities and who were willing to accept happy and safe over perfect, one of the themes I stress over and over here.

When I ask Benny what he remembers about that camp, it's funny. He doesn't remember us coming to camp when his inset came out in the lake or that he had to check BG before lunch and popsicles every day. He does remember zipping around the lake on the "banana boat," taking field trips to the local museums, and running around playing games until the end of every sweaty, dirty day. That was a terrific experience, and he went to that camp for a few years until we decided it was time for the next step.

Regular Sleepaway Camp

Growing up, I thought everyone went away to camp. My whole family spent time at what they now call residential camp. My dad, my sister and I, my husband, and our kids have had that experience. It wasn't until I got older and found that friends didn't go away from home for six or eight weeks every summer that I realized it was kind of unique.

I have friends who still can't believe we do this, diabetes or not. Don't we miss the kids? How do we have any family time? What do I do with myself while the kids are away for so long? What kind of parent ships their kids off for weeks at a time starting in elementary school?

I think if you've been to camp, it's easier to understand. There is an independence and confidence that comes from going away from home at a younger age in a supportive but challenging environment. Camp also taught me how to stack dishes like a pro, take a super quick shower, and do whatever job the "chore wheel" gave me that morning. Camp showed me who I was without my family and school friends right there. Who did I want to be? What decisions would I make? It truly shaped me into the person I am today.

My mother always jokes that the first year your child goes to camp, you cry when the bus pulls away. The second year, you cry when the bus comes back. At least I think she's joking.

Truly, that time away is great not just for the child but also for the parent. I like knowing who I am without my kids around. I like having extra time to work or organize photos or just not cook for anyone else. When camp starts, I can't wait to be alone and spend time with my husband. By the time camp ends, I can't wait for my kids to come home. It's a great break for everyone, and it makes me a better (and better rested) mom when my kids come back home.

Regular camp, though, is a much different – and more difficult – type of challenge for kids with type 1 diabetes. Here's a blog I wrote the first summer Benny went away to regular sleepaway camp in 2013.

> I pride myself on being pretty confident when it comes to my children and my decisions. They may not always be right or the best, but I'm usually pretty clear that they are the right and the best for us. But right now I'm doubting myself.
>
> We sent Benny to regular overnight camp.
>
> People without diabetes probably just shrugged, but I heard that gasp from the diabetes community. Sending kids to diabetes camp is a big deal for many parents. It often represents the first time a child has been away from home for a few hours, let alone overnight. It's staffed by doctors and nurses, and almost every staffer and counselor has type 1 diabetes. These people know what they're doing.
>
> Regular camp is different. Yes, they have medical staff, but there's no one specializing in type 1 diabetes.

Many of these people have never seen a pump before, or even if they're a school nurse, chances are they've never changed a pump site or filled a cartridge because parents come to school.

But this is my daughter's fourth year away at her camp. Every summer she comes home and reminds Benny that, "you can come with me when you're going into third grade." And I would just shrug and say, "We'll see." Well, guess who's going into third grade this fall? Yep, he wanted to go.

I've been working since January to make this happen, and I have to say, the camp is being great. We are all working hard to ensure a safe and fun experience. But I'm really, really nervous.

How nervous? That first year, Benny went away for just two weeks, common for the youngest group, and I woke up every morning at 4 a.m. in a cold sweat, convinced I had made the biggest mistake of my life and his life too. How could I have sent Benny away to "regular" camp? Didn't I know he had diabetes? Every bad scenario, big and small, ran through my brain. What if a low stopped him from having fun? Would the other kids make fun of him or exclude him? What if something really bad happened, and no one helped?

Remember that we didn't have a CGM until age 9, so the first year away at this camp, he was just using a meter. And there is no cell service in the area, so we never remote monitor. He uses the Dexcom receiver and puts away his phone.

He did just fine that first year, but I won't kid you – it took a lot of work. Benny had to be able to do all care by himself with supervision. I relied on the nurses to check in on him and make sure his sites look OK, and we kept the insulin at the infirmary, so he had to see them every couple of days.

The first year, they actually checked on him every night. Anyone in that age group who takes medication after dinner goes to the infirmary as a group. It turned out to be a good time – they get a golf cart ride and hang out in the air conditioning. Each night, they'd check his site and make sure he had insulin in his pump.

We learn each year and make improvements to the plan. The following year, he just checked in with the nursing staff when he needed insulin or ran out of supplies in his bag, which he carried everywhere. The very first year the staff helped him with food choices and with eyeballing carb counts. He didn't like that at all. (Who wants to have someone watch them eat?) So we've since come up with a few shortcuts and reminders to help him out.

Benny uses a camelback backpack at camp. It holds water, which is great for any camp, and he can have low supplies and anything else he wants to keep nearby on hand. In the cabin, we use plastic containers to hold juice boxes and crackers. You don't want anything messy or out of the wrapper – animals and bugs can be a problem! I also got him a bedside caddy that can be used on a bunkbed, so he could have his diabetes stuff right next to him at night.

We also put those day camp "action sheets" into the bag Benny carried around camp. Again, having our endo's input on what was needed to keep Benny safe at camp was extremely helpful. And having the doctor's signature on everything goes a long way to giving staffers peace of mind. As he got older, those papers were just kept at the infirmary, still on file if anyone had questions.

I admit, it would be tough to send my young child with T1D to a long-term residential camp without at least one nurse or doctor. While lows are important to watch out for, in my opinion, unchecked high BG and dehydration are the bigger worries. Those can lead to diabetic ketoacidosis (DKA) very quickly; you need someone who understands that. I have a hard-and-fast rule that they must call me if Benny throws up more than once in a six-hour period. They'd call anyway – any illness is taken seriously – but I want to be able to help troubleshoot what could turn into a serious situation.

This year is Benny's eighth at this sleepaway camp. I still wake up the first few mornings he's away freaking out and thinking I've made the worst decision ever. But I let him go because it's right for him. He loves this camp, and he's made incredible friends who keep in touch all year long.

You might be thinking, what if my kid doesn't want to go to camp? How do I know if it's right for them? This is a tough one. There are a lot of stories about kids taken to camp kicking and screaming who then didn't want to leave when camp was over! But camp isn't for everyone, and I'd hate for a parent to feel guilty or upset if their child doesn't go. I advise everyone to give it a try once.

Of course, there are other barriers to sending your child to camp. Cost is usually the biggest. Again, I know how lucky we are to be able to give our children this experience. There are scholarships for almost every camp and ways to fundraise. The Lion's Club is one group that usually awards diabetes camp scholarships; dig around for others. Many camps offer their own scholarships or at least installment plans.

Here's something Benny wrote at age 10 for a JDRF presentation all about camp:

> The best part of diabetes camp is the big dance.
> The big dance is the last night of camp, and I love it because I'm a party animal and I like to dance. If you don't want to dance or there's no one to go with, there's a movie option.
> I also like the zip line, swimming and the time we got to paint all over our bodies and had a competition between boys and girls to see who could cover a gigantic piece of paper first. Boys won.
> The worst part of diabetes camp is that it only lasts for a week.
> My advice to a new camper is to have fun and relax. The counselors make sure everyone meets each other. They are really fun.

On the first day, there can be a lot of waiting around. It can be boring. But tough it out because the fun is about to begin.

If you're new and feeling homesick, write a letter. It'll make you feel better.

I was scared the first time I went to camp. But Benjan Canadian (nickname) – my counselor – made me feel better just by being amazing. We had a lot of fun.

PMA means positive mental attitude. You get an older camper who's in the level right before staff, and they hang out with you. They may also send a letter home with you. I look at mine every time I think of camp. The letter makes me feel awesome, and I miss my older brother. Sometimes you get an older brother and an older sister. I got both last year. And if you're feeling down about your diabetes during the year, you can look at the letter and keep your PMA.

PMA. Every day.

ASK YOUR DOCTOR

- Is my child ready for diabetes camp, and how do I find one in our area?

- Can you provide extra prescriptions and/or supplies for sleepaway camp?

- What skills does my child need in order to go to "regular" day or sleepaway camp?

- What summer goals should we work on?

CHAPTER 13

Social Media Support

Benny said he was really thirsty. With a BG of 458, no wonder! That's way too high and not a number we see very often. I started to give a bolus, but the remote kept telling me it couldn't find the pump. "Oh yeah," Benny said. "That's because I don't have it on!" Why wouldn't it be on? I'd changed the insulin cartridge right before dinner – did I forget to give him the pump back? Where did I put it?

D o you share your diabetes mistakes on social media? What about your "wins?" Let's talk for a bit about social media and community. Not everyone is lucky enough to find support for diabetes in real life, but there is a thriving online diabetes community. You might be part of one of the hundreds of diabetes Facebook groups, some of which have tens of thousands of members. Or maybe you participate in a weekly Twitter chat or follow some T1D influencers on Instagram.

I think there's an argument to be made that we can get more out of social media when we share our mistakes and worries than when we only post when things are going "right." I know a lot of people love to share straight CGM lines and big and small victories, and that's great. I love to celebrate along with you! But over the years, I find I have more of an impact and get more support when I pull the curtain back and show what's not going right for us.

The first time I realized this was a scorching summer Saturday in 2010. Benny had just finished kindergarten and Lea fourth grade. It was 101 degrees in Charlotte. I took the kids out to lunch and then to a nearby splash pad. It was exactly what we needed, and we spent the afternoon inside at home, trying to beat the heat.

The afternoon blood sugar check was a shocker: 500 BG. An hour after a big bolus, Benny said he didn't feel well. At this check we got the dreaded "HIGH GLUCOSE" reading the meter gives you when the number is out of its range. No ketones, thankfully, but something was very wrong. The meter remote was across the room, so I asked Benny to take his pump out of the pouch he wears around his waist. That's when the problem became very clear. He had no pump to take out. Uh oh.

Even though the pump we used was waterproof, we usually took it off when Benny was in or around water. It wasn't the rough play. The insets stayed on just fine for that kind of thing, and the pump is durable. But Benny usually went low during swimming, and taking the pump off helped keep him steady.

Note that this definitely depends on the person. As Benny gets older and bigger, the energy he uses for swimming and water play has changed. When you think about a 5-year-old swimming, think how exhausted they get – they use their whole body every second! A 12-year-old is still very active but might be throwing a ball in the pool and hanging out for hours rather than swimming nonstop for 30 minutes. We found as he got older, we needed to increase the basal rate for a couple of hours after swimming if we'd disconnected for more than an hour.

As I said earlier, check with your endo about disconnecting a pump and/or adjusting the basal rates on a waterproof pump or pod. Many people have also found success using long-acting insulin along with the pump (also called "untethered) or even switching back to multiple daily injections for vacations or summer if your child swims a lot.

Whether your child swims for 10 minutes or 10 hours, you do need to put the pump back on. We had forgotten that part. As soon as I realized that, I immediately remembered what I had done. We'd taken off the pump and thrown it in my purse. It was still there, just blinking at me and dripping insulin. All that time I was giving Benny insulin using the remote meter, I'd really been bolusing my purse!

Once we figured that out, it wasn't a difficult fix. We clicked the pump tubing back into the inset, did a giant bolus, checked ketones (nope), and refilled Benny's water. I spent a moment wondering if I should wash my purse or just wipe it out. And if I'd ever get rid of the insulin smell. Ugh.

Fifteen minutes later I grabbed the meter to see if the insulin had started working. Yes, I know it was too soon, but I was nervous and anxious and … I dropped the meter. It slipped out of my hands onto the floor and cracked. I have backup meters, but this was the brand-new remote meter we'd only had for a month. After almost four years of pumping, we finally didn't have to reach into Benny's pouch to pull out the meter and could easily dose him while he slept. I didn't have to turn around in the car while my husband drove and dig around in Benny's car seat to bolus him for road trip car snacks. We loved that new meter. And now, it was all in pieces on my kitchen floor.

Talk about feeling like the world's worst diabetes mom. My kid was high because of my doofus forgetfulness. Our brand new amazing remote meter was in pieces. Surely no one was as horrible a mom as me.

I took my frustration to Twitter. If I tell you the responses were life-changing, I'm not sure that would be an exaggeration. This was back in 2010 when social media wasn't what it is today. I wasn't sure what I would get. Scorn? Judgment? Turns out, all I received was support.

@kellyemmaellis: oh no, simple mistake!! At least it can be easily corrected with pump and Benny had

been nice and active to take the edge off!!
@SweeterCherise: hugs! How's he doing?
@DMomBlog: It happens. You realized it and are
taking care of the situation. He'll be fine. ((hugs))
@Kate_Ireland123: diabetes is 24/7, you are not.
You can't be perfect all the time. It's not your fault, you
treated it, it's over :)
@PortblPancGrl: glad he's ok! And hope his BG gets
back to normal soon.

Other people had done this. Other people made it through.
They said I didn't have to be perfect and that Benny would be fine.
It's hard to describe how much better that made me feel. I was still
mad and frustrated, but I was no longer alone.

I think I was just as relieved to hear that Benny would be
OK – that this had happened before – as I was to see these other
women not judging me. Not shaming me. They didn't share the post
and invite others to pile on. Instead, they supported me. I didn't
know them, but they were willing to reassure me and lift me up.

Of course, Benny was fine. His blood sugar came down, and he
was safe and happy and thought the idea of bolusing my purse was
very funny. I called Animas, and they overnighted a new meter
remote. Ours was still in warranty (barely out of the box), so they
were fine with a quick replacement.

As you know by now, this was hardly our first mistake. But it
was the first time I remember admitting to one publicly. It was
incredibly freeing, and it led the way for me to share more mistakes
and missteps. We didn't have to wait long. Just a few months later, I
wrote about another fiasco in my blog.

We rarely check Benny's blood sugar between
dinner and bedtime. But last night, around 7 p.m.,
Benny said he was really thirsty. With a BG of 458, no
wonder! That's way too high and not a number we see
very often.

I started to give a bolus, but the remote kept telling me it couldn't find the pump. "Oh yeah," Benny said. "That's because I don't have it on!"

Why wouldn't it be on? I'd changed the insulin cartridge right before dinner – did I forget to give him the pump back? Where did I put it?

I jumped up and went to the kitchen while Benny looked around the family room. No pump anywhere. It wasn't in my purse this time. Trust me, after last time that was the first place I checked!

We'd had at least one time when Benny left his pump at home, having disconnected for a shower. In fact, that week he went one day without his meter, the next day without his pump, and on the third day, the nurse texted me that she was worried he was going to forget his pants! We always had a backup plan though; those safety nets had gotten us through before.

I tried to keep those reassuring thoughts in mind as Benny and I looked high and low. But I felt myself getting angry. Not at him, not even at diabetes. We've been having a pretty miserable January.

Benny had started getting migraines a few months earlier. We thought we had it under control after eliminating aspartame in the fall, but he'd already had three this month. Slade had rotator cuff surgery January 3rd, so my right-handed, very helpful husband was currently a lefty who could barely lift a fork. I'd also had some big deal changes at work. Losing an insulin pump just seemed like another thing to deal with before January would let us go.

By the way, losing diabetes pump stuff can happen whether you use a tubed pump or not. With the non-tubed pump, you still need the remote to give insulin. (Omnipod's is called a PDM, a personal diabetes manager.) So if you lose that, the background (basal) insulin will continue, but you can't give any more for high BG or for food. It's one reason Benny didn't want to switch to the pods. He knew he'd forget the separate PDM. But at least with the pods, the background insulin continues. Sigh. Everything's a trade-off. Why can't this be easier?

After searching for a few more frantic minutes, Benny and I decided to retrace our steps. He remembered putting the pump on during dinner, then taking a walk with his dad, and then playing with our neighbors across the street.

"Mom!" he shouted. "I remember! I took it off to play tackle football. But I didn't get tackled. I know where it is!"

Across the street in the dark we went. We found it right in Mr. and Mrs. J.'s yard, exactly where he left it – in the grass on their front lawn.

Benny and I had a good talk on the short walk home about better places to leave the pump, and whether it really needed to come off for front-yard football at all. We decided if he really wants to take it off, the mailbox or even the front door was probably a better choice than chucking it in the grass.

After a few moments of silence, Benny said, "I was really worried about losing it."

"Dude, I want you to be responsible, but we will always find or replace your pump."

Another pause. "But, Mom, I know it's really expensive."

Did you hear my heart break? Why does my 7-year-old need to worry or even know about this?

I said, "When it comes to diabetes, we will always, always, find a way to make it work. You don't have to worry."

Benny said, "OK!" He looked over and smiled at me, then sweetly said, "I really have to pee."

> Well, he was still really high. At least he made it
> back to our yard!

When I posted that story, I received nothing but support and "been there" from the diabetes online community. It was also one of the first times people shared that our lousy experience made them feel better. We all have those feelings of imperfection, not being good enough, and even some anger. Sharing them makes us all realize all of those reactions are totally normal.

It's been almost a decade since that post, and I still think the diabetes online community is different from most of the rest of the internet. It's still a place of support and a repository of incredibly valuable information. It's almost what we wish the internet would be for everything.

Of course, I got the idea for this book from someone being absolutely miserable to me online. But those experiences, thankfully, have been few and far between. Believe me, I realize that there are a lot of pitfalls out there, even within the diabetes community. Most of those, though, come from feeling like you're not measuring up, from only following people who want to share perfect numbers and flawless pictures. Don't let that staged perfection fool you.

Find people to follow and groups to participate in where you feel understood, where you feel trusted and lifted up. If you're not getting a benefit from social media, it's OK to step away, to mute a group or a "friend" or to follow those you trust. It's OK to delete an entire post if you want, or a comment thread, like I did with the rude troll who told me I really was the worst.

On Facebook, I'd be careful of enormous closed groups; start with a smaller local group. You can search T1D and your town to see if there is one. People tend to be nicer and more careful in their posts if there's a chance you might run into them at the JDRF Walk or even the grocery store.

On Twitter, a great place to find support is with the hashtag #DSMA. That stands for diabetes social media advocacy, and they have a weekly chat. But you can use the hashtag anytime to find support.

I hesitate to give more specifics here, because social media is always changing. But what doesn't change is the idea that we should try to use it to connect and support.

ASK YOUR DOCTOR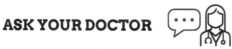

- What's the backup plan when the pump isn't working, we forget it or leave it somewhere, or we lose the pod controller?

- What's our plan for swimming or anytime we need to disconnect the pump?

- What's the plan for very high numbers? Should we have different correction factors for higher numbers?

- When should we check for ketones and how often?

CHAPTER 14

The Big Field Trip

Around 2 a.m. my phone buzzed with the Dexcom urgent low alarm. Benny was 55. Then he dipped down to the point where it just yelled LOW at me. I texted him. No response. ... How could I have allowed him to go on this trip? What kind of parent lets her child have a low blood sugar while he's 400 miles away?! That was it. He was never leaving the house again.

Fifth grade in our elementary school was a big deal. It's the oldest grade in the school, and the kids have more responsibility and privileges, and on Fridays they're allowed to walk the five or six blocks and hang out in our village green. Yes, we live in small-town America. There's even an honest-to-goodness soda shop!

The biggest milestone in fifth grade is the three-day trip to Washington, D.C. Benny had been looking forward to this for a long time.

They ask parents to chaperone, and there are so many volunteers that they have to institute a lottery. Because of Benny's diabetes, my husband was able to skip the lottery; he was already in as a chaperone. That changed when, a few months before the trip, Slade got a new job. He had to travel the week of the D.C. trip.

I thought about asking to go, but as a female chaperone for boys, it would get a little tricky. (The chaperones sleep in the same room.) Benny did not want me doing anything special, like pulling him out of the group or making the trip "different" for him in any way because of diabetes. I couldn't go book a hotel room for just him and me – part of the fun of this trip is staying in a hotel with your school friends. When you're 11 years old, doesn't that sound like the coolest thing in the world? Staying with your mom is not the same.

So, as usual, we had to figure out a backup plan. I spoke to the school, and we all agreed, if we found a willing chaperone, Benny could bunk with two other boys just like everyone else for the two nights of the trip. A school friend's dad who was also our neighbor seemed like a great choice. So I called up Mr. P. and took him out for coffee.

Mr. P. is a great guy. He's a stay-at-home dad, and Benny had spent many afternoons at his house. But that was the extent of their time together. It's tough to figure out exactly how much someone who knows your child but isn't very well versed in type 1 diabetes needs to know to keep everyone safe and happy.

Luckily, Benny was pretty self-sufficient at that point. We were operating under the "trust but verify" school of thought. He did all his school BG checking and insulin dosing himself but confirmed with a teacher just before lunch to make sure all was well. We didn't have a full-time nurse, and this was a compromise that kept everyone happy and Benny safe.

In fourth grade, that confirmation meant showing his teacher the blood sugar meter or Dexcom receiver, and by fifth grade, it was simply a thumbs up back and forth. At home, I still helped with a lot of Benny's management, but I knew he'd be OK with a responsible adult for a few days.

I decided I wouldn't train Mr. P. on glucagon. The principal knew enough about that, and he'd be in the room next door to this group. We came up with a plan, focusing less on perfection and more on safe and happy. Since Benny had Dexcom Share by that point, there was no need for him to verify his BG by showing it to anyone. I could see it and call him or the chaperone if needed. He would look at his blood sugar at mealtimes (at a minimum) and confirm with Mr. P. that he'd bolused – just a thumbs up was good enough for me. Each night, they'd repack his bag for the next day and make sure he had enough insulin in his pump for the night.

Benny carried his diabetes bag everywhere, and Mr. P. had backup supplies with him as well. I'm pretty sure the principal also had low supplies. They were definitely looking out for him.

Benny and I spoke separately about food – I knew this would be his biggest concern. He wasn't to the point yet where he could accurately carb count for new food, and there were at least two all-you-can-eat buffets on this trip. Dude likes to eat, and I wanted him to be able to dose well and not feel weird about the whole thing. I wanted him to enjoy some dessert, but I also didn't want him hanging off the chocolate fountain at Golden Corral!

Informed and with a plan, Benny went on the trip. The bus ride to D.C. and the first evening went great. Benny texted me with some dosing questions, and we checked in with each other right before bedtime. Then around 2 a.m. my phone buzzed with the Dexcom urgent low alarm.

Benny's BG was 55. Then he dipped down to the point where it just yelled LOW at me. I texted him. No response. I texted Mr. P. No response. I waited. I stayed calm. I imagined them treating the low, hearing my texts but very wisely deciding to treat before responding.

Then I imagined them ignoring everything. Or maybe all the low treatments had fallen out of the bag, or they'd left the bag somewhere. I imagined the little diabetes backpack all by itself on the steps of the Lincoln Monument. I imagined Benny and his friends scrambling around the hotel room looking for something, anything to bring up his blood glucose.

How could I have let him go on this trip? What kind of parent lets her child have a low blood sugar while he's 400 miles away?! That was it. He was never leaving the house again.

I took a deep breath and tried to think logically. If I called the principal's cell phone or had the hotel ring his room, he'd be up and in there in a moment, but it was 2 a.m. I decided calling him was a solid safety net but didn't want it to be my immediate option.

That Dexcom alarm gets pretty loud. There was no way all four people in that room could ignore it. I decided they were treating and that I would give it a little time. It had felt like hours, but when I looked back at my phone, it was really only about two minutes.

OK, I thought. Breathe. Sure enough, in 10 minutes, the Dexcom arrow turned around, and within 15 minutes, Benny's BG was 85. I waited a little longer and watched it slowly float up above 100. I went back to bed knowing that, despite the communication issue, my son was safe.

My phone blew up around 7 a.m. "Mom, why did you text? I just grabbed my Gatorade and drank it. I didn't even need to wake anyone up. Love you."

Our sleepover protocol has long been that if he wakes up to a Dexcom low alert, or if he wakes up and just feels low, to drink the Gatorade right away. We don't do that at home – I'll usually confirm via fingerstick and dose with a more specific amount of carbs, but on the road, by himself, this takes all the guess work out.

Mr. P. was horrified. He had texted a very sweet and panicked apology. Then he called me. He just hadn't heard my text. And he obviously didn't hear Benny's Dexcom alarm. We pieced together that Benny had heard it, woken up, and shut it right off as he treated. In his fifth grade brain, there was no need to wake anyone else up. He'd treated, and everything was fine.

I assured Mr. P. that, if needed, the Dexcom alarm would've woken them all up eventually. Even so, he was determined to sleep lightly the next night. I wasn't sure he'd ever sleep again.

The second day of the trip started off really well. In fact, the whole day was fine. That evening, though, Benny needed a little help. With my husband away, my daughter and I made plans to enjoy some time together. I got tickets to a Broadway show coming through town. We got dressed up, went out to dinner, and had a great time. At the start of the second act, my phone started buzzing. It was Benny. I excused myself and went into the lobby.

His blood sugar was pretty high, and he was trying to troubleshoot. The inset seemed to be working (no visible leaks at least), and he'd bolused for dinner, but was it enough? We talked it through and decided to give a little more insulin via the pump and check back in 45 minutes when the play would be over.

He called back in an hour; we were in the car inching out of the crowded city parking garage. His BG stayed pretty much where it had been. "I think I should take a shot," Benny said. I agreed; that was a great idea. Only problem: He'd never given himself a shot without us there. He was nervous.

My daughter had the solution. "FaceTime us! We'll talk you through it!" She pulled out her phone, and we joked and talked until he felt OK enough to do the shot.

I asked him if he wanted to change the inset as long as he had us on the phone, but he declined, saying he really thought he'd just under-bolused for dinner, which means he probably ate an enormous dinner and dessert and just didn't want to tell us. I didn't push. The important thing is that he called me for help and that he was troubleshooting. His blood sugar came right down and stayed steady all night. So it wasn't the inset anyway.

You might be thinking, why is this kid – who's had diabetes for more than eight years at this point – afraid of shots? It's actually a very common issue among kids who start pumps very young. We think we're doing them a favor by just switching to the pump insets and putting away the pens and syringes. I'm telling you: Learn from me and don't do that.

Being able to administer an insulin shot is a great adjunct tool to pumping. As I've mentioned, insets can get wonky. If you're not sure an inset it working, it's very helpful to be able to give a shot, change the inset, and move on. Insets can come off or just get knocked off (pods too), and being able to inject can save everyone a lot of stress.

Being able to see us took away a lot of that stress for Benny and helped him do that first independent injection. The rest of the trip passed with no issues. The next night was great, although Mr. P. probably didn't sleep much, and the kids came home the next day worn out from all the walking and excited about completing the fifth grade trip.

Benny hasn't looked back. That trip marked a huge turning point for his independence, self-care, and confidence. He still had a long way to go before he was ready for full self-care, but looking back, it was a milestone in his diabetes care. He knew when to ask for help, that he could ask for help and that he really could manage diabetes away from us. What a great way to end elementary school.

ASK YOUR DOCTOR

- In what situations might we need to use shots while on an insulin pump? Do we need an extra prescription for pens and/or syringes?

- What should my child's diabetes kit contain while on overnights and extended field trips?

- How should my child treat lows or have chaperones treat lows while not at home?

CHAPTER 15

Sports

About five minutes later, the low alert blared again.
Now I was worried. If he was low during a game, he
could mess up and forget a play. More importantly,
he could get hurt. I looked as closely as I could
from the sidelines. He looked fine. He was making
tackles. "What do we do?" I said out loud. I knew
what I wanted to do, I wanted to run onto the field
yelling, "My baby! My baby!" and carry him off.
Of course, Benny was now bigger than me, so that
would have been difficult, but I was willing to give
it a try.

Benny was never the kind of kid to pick a sport and stay with
it. That meant every couple of years, we were learning how
to navigate a new activity with diabetes. By now, you know that
means we messed up until we almost got it right.

Sports are tricky for most people with T1D because the body's
reaction can be unpredictable. Usually exercise will help bring blood
sugar down. But sometimes the drop comes much later. Sometimes
adrenaline and excitement will raise blood sugar. Different types of
exercise affect blood sugar in different ways. Weight lifting is not
the same as heavy cardio, like running. I'm hardly an exercise and
diabetes expert, but I can tell you our stories.

Benny's first sport was just being a toddler. You laugh, but that's some Olympic-level sprinting and energy bursts. Tough to manage, but we found that he would often go low a bit after playtime. A snack before nap helped a lot in those days. I was also the mom at the playground yelling, "Get back here and drink this juice!" or "You can't play anymore until you eat something!" Then I'd throw a cookie at him – always good for some weird looks at new playgrounds.

His first real sport was soccer. To call little-kid soccer a sport is a stretch, but we'll start there. It was really fun. Benny was about 5 years old when we started. Soccer was pretty easy – the games were short, and parents rotated bringing snacks for everyone.

The hardest part of soccer was navigating those snacks. When it was our turn, we'd provide fruit and water and maybe small granola bars. But other parents brought giant juice pouches, cookies, and chips. It was frustrating; these 6-year-olds just ran around for 15 minutes, do they really need 100 carbs right now?

We decided that rather than explain to everyone about type 1 diabetes, we'd just have Benny stick to water and bring the juice home for another time. Or he'd drink the juice and save the cookies. Over the course of the seasons, we did explain to some parents who asked about the insulin pump or saw us checking blood sugar. A few parents did switch to water, or lower sugar drinks, which was great. But we'd been at this for almost four years already, and I'd already started picking my battles of how much of diabetes to explain and to whom.

His next sport was touch football. My favorite story about that has nothing to do with diabetes; I wasn't even there when it happened. He was playing a game, and at a timeout he walked over to my husband. "My tooth feels funny," he said.

"The loose one?" Slade asked.

"Yeah." Then Benny pulled the tooth out and handed it over. "I gotta go back in."

I'm glad I wasn't there. I would have probably wadded the tooth in a tissue if I remembered at all to save it for the Tooth Fairy. Slade took a picture and proudly texted it to his brothers. Gross.

Benny played a little bit of basketball, which honestly, I hated for diabetes. He was in fourth grade by then, too old for me to hover all over him during games. But that was also the year we got the Dexcom CGM, so I was able to better keep an eye on things. This was pre-Share, so no cell phone blood sugar readings. I'd hold the receiver and sit in the stands. That was pretty cool. But basketball was still hard for us.

Often by the second quarter, Benny would start going low. He'd treat during timeouts; I don't remember him missing playing time. Mostly, his BG would be unpredictable a few hours later. We had just started to really figure out how to keep things steady when he changed his mind and went all in on baseball.

Baseball was the sport Benny played the most in elementary and into middle school. I love baseball for diabetes. It can be slow, and there are a lot of breaks and plenty of time to test blood sugar. From my blog:

> This will be Benny's third year playing baseball and his first with kid pitch. Our town's league has a really fun atmosphere. I'm a fan, mostly because it's not a sport where I worry too much about diabetes.
>
> Having said that, Benny went low about 15 minutes into his first practice. Dropping from a comfy 150 (arrows holding) to a 90 with double arrows down. He chugged a PowerAde, sat down for a few minutes and went back in. His blood sugar never went above 80 for the rest of the practice (or for about an hour after). No big spike later either. He needed that drink!

My favorite baseball memory has nothing to do with the game. Benny is always very open about diabetes. One day in the dugout, a friend asked him about his insulin pump. Instead of just explaining it, Benny took out the pump and let his friend dose him! I heard about this much later, after everything was over.

We saw the boys all crowding around something in the dugout. I assumed it was a bug or a booger, not my son's insulin pump! Benny tested his blood glucose, then showed the other boy how to enter the value into the pump, get the recommended dose, and then manually enter that recommendation. I found this out about two innings later when I did a regular check of the CGM. Again, no Share yet, so we hung the Dexcom receiver on the dugout wall. I'd go over and look every once in a while; of course, it would alarm if we really needed to take action. That's when Benny told me his friend had dosed him.

What?! After I got the whole story, I found the boy's mom and explained what had happened. I didn't want him going home and telling his family who-knows-what about what he thought he'd done. And I told Benny that while it's great to educate, it's probably not the best idea to hand over his pump to anyone else. It was that weird parental mix of surprised, worried, and also a bit proud.

Every new sport and every new team required education. Our experience has only been up until middle school, so the intensity is not as strong as it may become. Certainly high school and college sports will require more work all around.

We always made sure coaches knew what they needed to. Often, Benny wasn't the first kid they'd coached with T1D. Almost always, they were willing to learn whatever they needed to make the sport fun and safe for everyone.

Our only unpleasant moments came from referees and umpires, usually because the timing can be rushed. This is where you really need the coach on your side. No ref wants to hear from a parent two minutes before a game about an insulin pump or a medical ID. I'd strongly suggest you go over these issues with your coach ahead of time to avoid unpleasant attention or delays at game time.

Football came along in seventh grade. Benny handled practices pretty well – sometimes he'd go low overnight, but we worked together to figure out better basal rates, etc. Games were a little trickier.

We had one terrible high that season. Benny had some pump issues at school; he'd been troubleshooting, but he started the game higher than his usual range and came out just before the half at 400. Sure enough, his pump site was leaking, so he definitely wasn't getting the insulin he needed.

High blood sugars can be even more dangerous during sports and exercise. As I've mentioned, ketones are acids that build up when your body can't break down glucose and instead starts to burn fat for energy. Playing sports and being very active will burn more fat and produce more ketones. Benny needed to come out of the game and get insulin and fluids into him, quickly.

He motioned me over to the sidelines. "What do I do?" I told him I thought a shot was the best idea. "In front of all these people?" I told him no one would notice if we didn't jump around and call attention to it. He hiked up his jersey, gave himself a shot, and went back to chugging water. He did sit out the third quarter, but he was feeling well enough to go back in before the end of the game. They still got creamed, but I'm counting that as a win.

The low was harder – for me. Benny played defensive tackle, and Slade and I were both watching from the sideline. Suddenly our Dexcom alarms started going off. We checked and both said, "Low." What? The coaches and assistants know to make sure Benny looks at his Dexcom or does a fingerstick before the start of the game and at each quarter. Surely that low was a misread or a compression low, where pressure on the sensor causes abrupt and false low readings. We agreed it couldn't be right – he was playing right in front of us and doing great! Then we lost the signal.

About five minutes later, the low alert blared again. Now I was worried. If he was low during a game, he could mess up and forget a play. More importantly, he could get hurt. I looked as closely as I could from the sidelines. He looked fine. He was making tackles.

"What do we do?" I said out loud. I knew what I wanted to do. I wanted to run onto the field yelling, "My baby! My baby!" and carry him off. Of course, Benny was now bigger than me, so that would have been difficult, but I was willing to give it a try.

Slade and I looked at each other. He knew what I wanted to do. He gave me that "stay calm" look I've come to know very well over the years. I made a mental deal with myself – I'd wait five minutes, then I'd grab the assistant coach and say something. I wouldn't make a huge fuss. I'd stay calm. But a low alert can't really be ignored.

Five minutes ticked by, and I second-guessed myself. What if it was a wrong reading? Maybe his pads had shifted causing a compression low? But it didn't look like that on the graph. It looked like a genuine "can we please just stop this football game and throw some juice down this kid's throat?!" low.

Just then, Slade tapped me, and I looked up from the graph on my phone. Benny had his helmet off and was trotting over to the bench. He sat down and drank a Gatorade. I watched him with relief. We were across the field, so I couldn't hear anything, but I saw the coach came over and check on Benny, give him a reassuring pat, and let him sit and recover. A little while later, he went back into the game. There were only a few minutes left at that point.

After the game, Benny told us he'd actually chugged two Gatorades. He finished the game with an 85 BG. Whew!

I told him that I wanted to run onto the field and save him. He was mortified just thinking about it. But we talked it out. I shared the plan I'd made in my head about quietly alerting an assistant coach or somehow getting him attention without making a spectacle of things. He wasn't thrilled but agreed that was the safe plan.

Most people I know who are successful with sports and diabetes have taken the time to make plans, to keep track of how their bodies react. It's not perfect, but over time, you can figure out how certain types of exercise will affect blood sugar.

JDRF has a terrific guide on exercise management in type 1 diabetes. They help with guidelines on glucose targets for and effective exercising with T1D, as well as nutritional and insulin dose adjustments to prevent exercise-related fluctuations in blood sugar. Learn more at https://www.jdrf.org/t1d-resources/peak/.

I think it comes down to education over and over again, for the person with diabetes, the family, the team, the coach, and the officials. It can take a lot of time and effort, but when you love a sport, it's worth it.

Benny is now deciding whether he wants to stay with football or try yet another new sport. This time, it's wrestling. And he's been doing more targeted workouts with a mix of cardio and strength training. So, for us, the diabetes sports learning will continue.

ASK YOUR DOCTOR

■ How do you recommend we plan for sports? Would it be helpful to track blood sugars or look at CGM readings? If yes, for what time periods and for how long?

■ What are the best treatments for lows during games or practices? Should we have a different plan later in the day or overnight on heavy activity days?

■ Should we check for ketones more often during sports or restrict activity when my child's BG is over a certain level?

■ Do you have any recommendations for – or cautions against – dietary changes for certain sports?

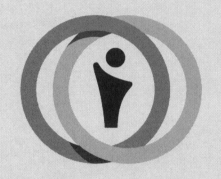

CHAPTER 16

Independence and Guilt

I dropped them off at the party and went 10 minutes away to Super Target. Hey, 10 minutes is a big step! They made it about 45 minutes into the two-hour party without calling me. My phone buzzed. "Mom," Lea said. "Benny doesn't look right. I think you need to come back." I looked at my cart. I looked at my watch. I'm not proud, but my first thought was, "Can I make it through the checkout line?"

Let's talk about independence. Letting go. This is going to be an easy chapter, right? After all it's so easy to let our kids go – diabetes on board doesn't add any stress to an already difficult transition.

Hahahahahahahah. OK.

As Benny got older, we encouraged him to be a "big kid" and check his own blood sugar and use his pump at preschool, always with supervision. At home, I still did almost everything for him. We felt that was a good trade-off for where he was with skills and readiness. We're talking about when he was 5 years old. I mean, I was still tying his shoes half the time!

Kindergarten took a lot of work, but our school was very supportive. At the time, Benny was the only child with type 1. I still went on every playdate, stayed at every birthday party, and felt a bit like a diabetes shadow.

Then we had the snow day.

We live in North Carolina, where any snow cancels school and empties grocery store shelves. When Benny was in first grade, we had a beautiful snowfall, a couple of inches of kid heaven. He and Lea begged me to let them go sledding down our street with friends. By themselves.

I loaded both kids up with juices boxes and granola bars. I talked to them about what would happen if Benny didn't feel well or thought he was going low. They promised me they'd stay on our block. They'd knock on the nearest door if they needed help. I gave them one hour and sent them out into the snow.

I lit a fire and tried to enjoy my quiet house. But after 30 minutes, I started to worry. Of course I was already worried about Benny, but then the wheels started turning about Lea. Had she stayed with her brother? Was I a terrible mom for making her play with him and watch him this way? Would she resent all of this when she was older? Would it make her worry more about him and create an unhealthy situation that way?

The diabetes worries took over after that. After 40 minutes, I was sure Benny was face down in the snow. I was arguing with myself about whether to pull on my boots and head out when the phone rang.

It was Benny, just a few houses away, asking me to pick him up. His blood sugar was normal; he was just worn out. Lea had walked him inside and went back out to play. The kids had a great time. They were proud of themselves, and most importantly, Benny was fine. Eventually, my heart stopped pounding.

After that, we started letting Benny play by himself at friends' homes. Take your meter; take a juice box and a snack. We tried a few different bags, even clipping the meter to his belt. The real solution for several years was his bike. He put a sporty little bag on the bike. It didn't look different from anyone else's, and everything fit. Now, he could not only visit friends who lived several blocks away, but also carry anything he needed in a little black bike bag that didn't look special or different, but meant independence, freedom, and a not-so-worried mom.

We set up a routine. He would call me with blood sugar numbers and let me know what he was eating. This had the added advantage of letting me know what my neighbors serve as after-school snacks. It is unbelievable. I'm looking at you neighbor who leaves a box of donuts on the counter. Or you Mrs. B. with your oatmeal cookie sandwiches.

Honestly, we usually let him eat what everyone else was having as long he covered for it. A lot of these kids were picky eaters who left food untouched and seemed to live on air. Benny has never been that kid. One neighbor even called me to tell me how much they liked having Benny over for dinner. "He loves everything I cook!" she said.

We made a rule: You can't get "in trouble" for diabetes stuff. Forget to check? Leave your meter somewhere? Just tell me, and we'll figure it out; no yelling or punishment. Dealing with diabetes is tough enough; we need Benny to know he can come to us with any issue. We'll deal with it and move on, even if I'm freaking out on the inside.

When Benny turned 8, I decided I would take the big step and start leaving him at birthday parties. Lea was invited along with him to one of our neighbor's parties. That seemed like a great test case. She could be a second set of eyes and call me if they needed anything. My friends knew just enough about diabetes to keep things safe. So I dropped them off at the party and went 10 minutes away to Super Target. Hey, 10 minutes is a big step!

They made it about 45 minutes into the two-hour party without calling me.

My phone buzzed. "Mom," Lea said. "Benny doesn't look right. I think you need to come back." I looked at my cart. I looked at my watch. I'm not proud, but my first thought was, "Can I make it through the checkout line?"

I told her to have him check blood sugar and treat if he was low. He was, and they did. Then I checked out of the store as fast as I could and headed back. Yes, I stayed and went through the checkout line.

We never were able to figure out how to plan and dose for bounce house, high-activity birthday parties. He'd start off on the high side – after a snack that we didn't cover – then dip down low enough that we'd have to treat and never with good timing to use the birthday cake we knew was coming for the low treatment. Then later in the day, we'd see some high numbers. A CGM ultimately made those days easier, but by then, bounce house parties were few and far between.

Our ventures into independence continued, and around age 10, I started worrying a bit about burnout. From my blog in 2015:

> We'd been very lucky. Benny was never shy about diabetes. He enjoys his freedom, and he takes care of himself, granted with some reminders. Of course, at this age, when we were together, he still wanted me to help out a ton when he was home. Why do all kids become incompetent at EVERYTHING when their mother is in the room?
>
> My friends who've been through the teen years talk about burnout and warn me about expecting him to do too much at a young age. We help a lot at home with site changes and BG checks when he wants. At the same time, I think he'd be insulted if I told him he couldn't or shouldn't take care of himself at school or when he's away from home. So we walk a fine line and try to take our cues from Benny as he changes and gets older.
>
> Here's something that worked really well for us to help that independence/burnout equation balance

out. Benny goes to "regular" sleepaway camp for almost a month each summer. It's not a diabetes camp, but they have a great medical staff. We all spend a lot of time each year working to make sure Benny can have a safe and fun time away. It's almost four weeks where he does every blood sugar check, every pump inset and CGM sensor change, fills the cartridges, etc. He loves this camp, and he thinks it's been worth all the work to go. (His older sister is there too.)

When Benny came home after the third year – at age 10 – I had a funny idea. He'd done an amazing job (objective opinion!), with only a couple of bad lows and highs. Overall, he'd kept his blood sugar in a really good range. But I knew it was a lot of work and a lot of brain power. So I made him an offer: "How about a diabetes-free day?" I asked.

The next day, Benny didn't have to think about diabetes once. We did all the BG checks, all the carb counts, everything. I wouldn't even tell him the numbers. It was fun, easy, and he loved it. After taking care of himself by himself (with supervision) for almost a month, I could tell he really enjoyed this kind of pampering. It reminded me of how it was back when he was first diagnosed, at 23 months, before he could do anything. And it was a reminder of how far we've come.

The next morning, it was back to normal. We told Benny he could ask for another "free day" whenever he wanted. So much of diabetes is mental. I can't imagine the brain power, energy, and attitude it takes to manage type 1 every day, and I have great respect for the adults who do it. Right now, we make a good team. I want Benny to know that kind of help is always there.

Do you think he'll come home for a "free day" when he's 30?

Another idea that has worked very well for us is having a quick talk at the beginning of each school year. We decide what, if anything, we want to change. As Benny gets older, he has more ideas and more input.

In kindergarten, we just decided to get through the year, logging every BG check and every pump dose. First grade, he wanted to buy lunch at school; we decided once a week was a good start for that. By fifth grade, he would check and bolus without anyone looking over his shoulder. Our compromise there was that he had to let his teacher know insulin had gone in. A discreet thumbs up before lunch took care of that.

For middle school, we agreed he could check in with the nurse or an adult only when he had an issue. We also decided that I would text him 20 minutes before lunch to remind him to bolus. He really likes that and asks me to continue every year so far, even as he's about to start high school.

Talking these ideas out doesn't mean school will be perfect, but it helps for everyone to know what the expectations are. Letting your child weigh in on age-appropriate diabetes decisions is vital to help them learn and process what they need to do. It also goes a long way to turning mistakes into learning and improving moments. In our case, we're able to show Benny how far he's come.

Like most diabetes parents, though, I feel a lot of guilt. I want to share something that has helped me with that. It's also helped me continue to let go even when I want to pull Benny back.

A few years ago, my local JDRF chapter hosted a retreat called "Women of Type 1." It was for women and teen girls with type 1 and moms of kids with type 1. They asked me to come and speak. I don't have type 1, and I don't have a girl with type one in my family. But my work on the podcast and being part of this community for so long sparked an idea.

I created a talk called "She Just Doesn't Get It" for the teens and moms. After a short presentation, I split the groups. The teens went next door with Lauren, a college student and type 1 herself. The moms stayed with me and a pediatric endocrinology nurse.

Then the separated groups answered the same questions. These were fill in the blanks, including:

- It drives me crazy when she _____.
- If I think about what her day must be like, it makes me feel _____.
- I admire her because _____.

The moms talked about admiring their daughters' strength, worrying about them being on their own, and admitted sometimes feeling like they hovered or nagged too much. The teens talked about being grateful and admiring their moms' strength, even though they said their moms did tend to hover and nag too much. There was a lot of laughter and some tears.

We brought the groups back together; I shared the moms' responses, and Lauren shared the teens' responses. When she read, "When I think about her day it makes me feel guilty," she started tearing up. I heard sniffling and saw nods all over the room. These teens feel guilty. Almost every single one of them. Guilty that diabetes makes their parents worry, that it takes up time and money and takes away from family and fun time.

Some of the moms were shocked. They shared that *they* felt guilty. Guilty for not being able to take away the burden of diabetes, for not doing more to help, for knowing that their daughters might not feel well while they themselves felt fine. Many thought they had shielded their kids from knowing how much diabetes takes. But the kids know.

We don't have to tell them. They just know.

It was a tough moment but a great one. We talked through guilt – how it implies that we feel we are at fault, that we've done something wrong, that we're a burden to someone else. How sharing that feeling can help lift that weight, giving the other person a chance to say, "Let me carry that load. Let me share your burden and lift you up," to say, "We aren't perfect, but we love you, and we'll do anything we can do help you through this."

I heard later that some of the moms called it a breakthrough moment. There was one teen who hadn't talked to her mom about how she felt about diabetes in two years. After the session, she opened up. (Surprise! She told her mom that sometimes she hates it.) I don't imagine we "fixed" anything. But that wasn't the point.

I'm so grateful to have helped nudge along the conversation. Because when we release those feelings, it's the first step in relieving them. I don't imagine we'll ever really separate guilt and diabetes. But it's easier to let it go, just a bit, when we do it together.

ASK YOUR DOCTOR

- Do you have any advice for birthday parties? What about activity and high-carb treats like birthday cake?

- What skills does my child need to manage a party or solo playdate?

- Do you recommend counseling for guilt and unspoken issues around diabetes that can take a huge mental toll?

- Where can I find a local counselor for me or for my child?

CHAPTER 17

Help From a Spouse or Partner

Here's something I found interesting. Our opposite schedules made it easier for me to not expect perfection – because I wasn't delivering it. If I wanted to skip baths at night because I was tired, I couldn't be angry when Slade called to tell me he had to come back home because he forgot to put Lea's shoes on one morning before they went to day care. That one's still pretty funny.

When I think about the diabetes parenting differences between my husband and me, my mind drifts to our linen closet. Specifically, to the towels.

When I first met my husband, Slade, he was adamant that the towels be folded a certain way. His mother had raised five boys, and she had insisted on order and cleanliness. Bless her. Slade always folded his towels into flat thirds. Hand towels, bath sheets, kitchen towels. His closets were orderly and calm.

My towels were generally folded however I felt like arranging them while distractedly watching TV. I experimented with rolling them (I saw it on a show), but for the most part, they were stacked in wobbly towers without much rhyme or reason. If you had looked at our linens, I'm not sure you would have predicted our marriage would last.

After 21 years of wedded bliss (right, sweetie?), we're still together. I'd argue the same properties that keep our marriage strong can be applied to type 1 diabetes parenting. But a happy home – and a neat closet – doesn't mean both partners do everything the same way. Different parenting styles can actually help in the long run. You just have to let them.

When Benny was diagnosed, we reacted very differently. Slade sprang into action around our house. He made Excel spreadsheets of foods and carbs. He bought a food scale, so we could weigh and measure everything Benny ate. He kept incredible blood glucose and dosing logs on a yellow legal pad in the kitchen.

I looked for support. I wanted to talk to people who had children with type 1, who were adults with type 1. I turned to blogs for information and inspiration. I tackled the nitty gritty tasks, but I was more interested in the big picture.

As the years went on, we continued to develop our own styles. I have always liked to do more for Benny, while Slade pushes him to do more for himself. If we start a new piece of technology, Benny and I usually sit down together to start it up. Slade asks Benny to walk him through what it is and show him how it works later on.

We both agree on what our long-term goals are as parents: We want both of our children to be confident, independent, and responsible. We've learned that our different styles will get us there.

Of course, unlike many parents, we took on the diabetes parenting tasks very equally from day one. Remember that I was working in early-morning radio when Benny was diagnosed, and Slade was spending almost every night at our restaurant. You can't interrupt a live broadcast with insulin dosing questions, and you can't expect a hot dinner order to wait while the chef takes a call about bedtime blood sugar.

Here's something I found interesting. Our opposite schedules made it easier for me to not expect perfection – because I wasn't delivering it. If I wanted to skip baths at night because I was tired, I couldn't be angry when Slade called to tell me he had to come back home because he forgot to put Lea's shoes on one morning before they went to day care. That one's still pretty funny.

Diabetes leaves less wiggle room for mistakes, of course, but you get the idea. If I over-treated a low blood sugar, resulting in a boomerang high, how could I be upset if he miscalculated the breakfast carbs? We knew we could trust each other to keep the kids safe and happy, even if the daily routine sometimes seemed chaotic.

We've worked hard to have a sense of humor and a realistic attitude about type 1 diabetes; we're trying to pass that along to Benny. Slade has truly done some heavy lifting: When he was younger, Benny liked to be held upside down sometimes to change his inset. I never once even tried. Some things are just for dads!

There are quite a few studies about dads and diabetes care, usually about how they aren't very involved and what that does to health outcomes. Of course, it's a stereotype that mom is always the primary caregiver and that dad is just earning a living and providing health insurance. While that's slowly changing, the studies agree that it's better for kids with chronic conditions to have involved and educated parents.

We also need to take a moment to recognize the single moms and dads raising kids with T1D on their own. That's an incredibly tough job.

Over the years, I've met many burned-out parents who just want a little bit more help from their partners. If that's you, what can you do?

Talk about it out loud. I started dating my husband in 1995, and sometimes I still forget he can't read my mind. We have to talk these things out. Sit down together, without your child, and articulate what's on your mind. Tell your partner how you're feeling. Tell them what you need. Even if it's "just" learning to change a cartridge or call the insurance company, they can help.

Then, and this is the hard part, you have to listen. Is your partner worried they won't manage your child's diabetes "correctly" and will somehow hurt the child? Are they worried you'll get mad if they mess up? Why aren't they pitching in more? Quite often, the spouse doing less might not feel welcome to do more. They're afraid you'll think they'll do it wrong.

If your partner truly doesn't understand the basics of insulin dosing, checking blood glucose, or using a pump or CGM, it's time to teach them. Depending on your child's age, consider getting them involved in teaching mom or dad. It's also a fun way for you to see how much your young child really knows. If your child is older, I'd still recommend this. Parents can always give kids a break if needed or if they're ill. You can't do that if you don't know how.

Of course, there are troubling cases of partners who don't want to learn and don't want to be "bothered." That's a different story altogether. It's rare, but it happens. While overall it's that partner who is missing out in the long run on a closer relationship and on time with their child, in the meantime, the other partner is getting exhausted and burned out. This is the time when an in-real-life community is vital. Lean on other parents of kids with T1D or friends who can help. None of us can do this alone.

With or without a supportive partner, I'd also highly recommend a family diabetes camp weekend or a diabetes conference. Many have sessions on this particular topic, and some have meetups or sessions just for moms or just for dads. Sometimes just hearing someone else's story can make a big difference.

Remember back in Chapter 8 when Benny only wanted Slade to do his Dexcom insertions? I was a little insulted. I shared that with Slade, and we talked about how, for some reason, it was the right thing at the time. I felt a little silly for being possessive about a diabetes chore, but it made sense because I had already done so much. And it made sense to let it go. Benny had confidence his dad would do a great job on a nerve-wracking insertion.

I just took a look in our linen closet. After living together all this time, the towels are folded in thirds, but the stacks are wobbly, and the calm order I remember from Slade's apartment isn't there. But it's a compromise of different styles that get the job done.

Of course, parenting a child with type 1 diabetes isn't exactly like folding towels or organizing a linen closet, but the idea is the same. You may disagree on whether to do a trifold or a deep fold or even that cool rolling method and whether to stack by color or size. As long as everything's clean and you know where to find it, why find fault?

Like mine, your partner probably already showed how they care about your child in different ways than you before diabetes came into your lives. As long as your child is safe and happy, embrace that difference. Knowing there's more than one management style can be a gift. In the long run, your child will be stronger, smarter, and more resourceful.

ASK YOUR DOCTOR

- Are there any local groups that provide support for spouses within families touched by type 1?

- Are there caregiver training opportunities for spouses or other family members who may not have received training at diagnosis or who need more education now?

- Do we have diabetes family camps in our area? What about diabetes family conferences?

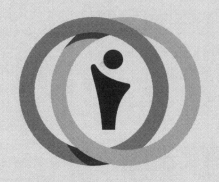

CHAPTER 18

Hulk Smash

Diabetes is frustrating and maddening, but I rarely
lose my cool or raise my voice in front of Benny. And
when I did, you'd think it would be about something
important like dosing or school accommodations
or even ordering supplies. Nope. I lost my s**t over
a sticker.

L et's talk about diabetes and frustration. And anger. When
Benny was very young, he didn't understand that his moods
were affected by his blood glucose levels. That makes sense; it's
hard for toddlers to articulate how they feel, even without diabetes.
My daughter never said, "I think I have an ear infection," when
she was in preschool. Instead, if she was in pain or uncomfortable,
she'd refuse to sleep or try to hit us. We caught on pretty quickly.

Benny was very similar in preschool when his blood sugar
was high. Like a lot of people with T1D, high blood sugar usually
makes him grumpy, quick to anger, and a bit unreasonable. Not
that a 3-year-old is reasonable to begin with, but you know what
I mean. It wasn't until about age 4 or 5 that we were able to start
working on a few strategies to help. One of the best involved
the Hulk.

The Marvel Cinematic Universe (MCU), as they call the
superhero movies based mostly on the Avengers comics, has been

a huge, fun part of my family's life. We've seen every MCU movie together up to this point. Lea's favorite character is Iron Man, and mine is Captain America. But Slade and Benny are Hulk fans – Slade because he watched the 1970s TV show with his mom, and Benny, in part, because of diabetes.

We started telling Benny that he was a lot like the Hulk when his blood sugar was high and he felt angry and mean. But unlike the Hulk's alter-ego Dr. Bruce Banner, we said, he could learn to control the big green guy.

We started by having him recognize that he was high – of course we'd test first – and then he'd work on removing himself from the situation. He could go to his room and beat up a stuffed animal or yell into a pillow. He could sit quietly with me and color and drink water and be mad. But he couldn't "release the Hulk" on other people. It wasn't perfect, but it helped him process what was going on in language he could understand.

The analogy got even better in the last Avengers movie. But before I can tell you about that, I have to admit, there are times when I have my own "Hulk smash!" moments with diabetes.

Diabetes can be frustrating and maddening, but I rarely lose my cool or raise my voice in front of Benny. And if I did, you'd think it would be about something important like dosing or school accommodations or even ordering supplies. Nope. I lost my s**t over a sticker.

Benny was going to a sleepover at a friend's lake house. Of course, they'd be swimming. I imagined they'd spend most of the evening in and out of the water, which was basically in this kid's backyard.

If you use diabetes gear, like a pump or a CGM, you know that it can be difficult to get everything to stay on in the hot weather or in the water. At that time, none of the overlays we'd tried had worked well on Benny's skin. He was just a few weeks into using the new Dexcom G6 system, and I was worried about losing the sensor and the more expensive transmitter.

I had a few overlays in the diabetes supply cabinet but only one with a Dexcom cutout. I gave it to Benny and walked out of the room, expecting to come back and help him in just a moment. Instead, I came back to him chatting happily with Slade while he distractedly placed the overlay.

Some of these sticky patches are really easy to mess up; they don't go on smoothly without time and effort. Of course, Benny wasn't putting in the extreme care I use to roll them on, and the overlay got completely squished. He pulled the mess off his arm and mashed it into a ball. To him, no big deal, it just wasn't working out.

To me at that moment? A disaster. Absolute catastrophe.

I heard myself hollering at him, as loud as I ever have: "What were you thinking?! That was the last one!!" I didn't even sound like myself.

Benny and Slade looked at me as though I had lost my mind. I can't remember another time when I yelled at my son about diabetes. In fact, we have a rule that you can't get in trouble because of diabetes. I saw in Benny's eyes that I'd scared him. Honestly, I'd scared myself.

Benny didn't say a word. He just went into his room and closed the door. Slade looked at me. "What was that about?"

It wasn't about the stupid overlay. You know that. It was all my fears about inconvenience, about Benny having to stop while his friends were playing in the lake, about having to call to replace supplies, about all the time and effort and worry about diabetes just building up until it had to come out. Unfortunately, it came out in a way that hurt the person I was trying to protect.

I took a deep breath, knocked on Benny's door, and went in to talk. I reassured him he hadn't done anything wrong. I tried to explain, but I think he filed it under "mom just worries" and moved on.

To be honest, I don't remember how this story ends. I have no idea if Benny found something else in our cabinet to put over the Dexcom. I'm not even sure if the Dexcom stayed on! I do remember he had a great time at the party. I was also grateful later that summer when we found StayPut Medical patches. Finally, something easy to put on that worked for Benny's skin. I think I ordered 5,000. (Just kidding! Maybe.)

There are times, though, when nothing really works, and T1D just gets the best of you. One night last year, Benny did an inset change, and it hurt more than usual. Even worse, it didn't work. He needed to do a second one, and that hurt as well. Unfortunately, it was one of those double days when he needed to change his Dexcom sensor as well.

The Dexcom hurt even worse. I don't know if he hit a nerve or muscle, but it hurt bad enough to make him curse out loud. I didn't mind that – we'd been letting him use "potty" words for inset changes and diabetes frustration since he was tiny. Then he burst into tears.

At that point, Benny was 13, bigger than me, and cried so rarely that I couldn't remember the last time he'd teared up. That night, he sobbed his heart out about how hard diabetes can be. What could I say? I don't have the same struggles, and more importantly, I can take a break. Of course, I will always worry about my children, but he will always have diabetes.

I hugged him and told him it was great to let it out. I tried to be reassuring, but mostly I just listened and sat with him. After a while, he said he felt better, got up, and did the Dexcom. He carried on and managed another day with the burden of diabetes. I admit that I felt a bit helpless. Sure, I gave him "mom" support, but I couldn't give him what I'd consider "real" diabetes support – the kind he gets at camp or from friends with T1D.

Amazingly, a few days later, we were scheduled to have dinner with some of those friends. I'd met Rodney Miller when he was a guest on my podcast. As the founder of Bolus and Barbells, he brings together people with type 1 diabetes and a passion for resistance training. Rodney and part of the group were passing through Charlotte on their way to a Bolus and Barbells event in Wilmington, North Carolina. When I saw him mention it on social media weeks earlier, I reached out to set up a dinner.

It was amazing – no talk of diabetes, just a bunch of guys eating barbecue and goofing around. Colt Scott (who later competed on "American Ninja Warrior") was there along with some local T1D friends who'd come for fun. They joked around with Benny about how he was going to be taller than all of them. (At 13, he was already 5 feet, 9 inches.) We took pictures, and I tried not to be too embarrassing.

The camaraderie of that night didn't cancel out the anger and pain of Benny's experience just a few nights before. It's not as though suddenly diabetes was any easier. But knowing that Rodney (who can pull a truck) and a ninja like Colt probably wince when they put on a new inset or CGM makes you feel a bit less alone, as does knowing it's OK if your mom doesn't really get it, because there are people out there who do.

Let's finish up that Hulk analogy I started earlier. Heads up – minor spoilers for "Avengers: Endgame" ahead.

There is a scene early in "Endgame" when the Hulk appears but in a completely new way. It seems that Dr. Banner has figured out a way to embrace his Hulk side, and the two are at peace. I wanted to stand up and cheer when I saw "Professor Hulk" on screen. You see, that's my hope for Benny.

He can't take diabetes and pretend it's somebody else. He can't take his bad moods and his highs and his lows and push them off on "the other guy" because all of that is truly a part of who he is. If Benny is able to embrace the side of him that he sometimes wants to reject, he'll be that much stronger.

■ What signs of mood changes should I look for when my child has high or low blood sugar? Do you have any advice on how to explain this to them and how to help them through it?

■ Are there local diabetes counseling resources available for families and/or specifically for kids and teens with type 1?

■ What's a good way to connect with other people who know what we're going through? Can you recommend separate resources for parents and for kids?

CHAPTER 19

Problem-Solving

"Mom. I left my medical bag with all my insulin
and everything in Greg's dad's car. I don't have any
insulin left in my cartridge, and I'm really high.
What do I do?" Even as my sleepy brain struggled
to read the text, my heart sank. We'd talked in
advance about taking his medical bag on the fishing
trip but being careful not to leave it in the sun all
day and about not dropping his cell phone in the
water. We had not talked about forgetting the bag
that held *all* of his insulin.

L ast summer I attended a session about teens with type 1
diabetes by the incredible Jill Weissberg-Benchell. She's a
certified diabetes educator, holds a doctorate in psychology, and
gives a great presentation about parenting a child with T1D . One
thing she said really stood out. She talked about watching for
signs of maturity, that your child really is making progress. One
of those signs, she said, is problem-solving.

I wanted to jump up and cheer.

We weren't messing everything up! What a relief. I've often
wondered if Benny is learning from all of these mistakes along
with us. That summer, I found out he was.

Just a few weeks earlier, my husband and I had taken a dream vacation. We decided to celebrate our 20th wedding anniversary with a trip to Monte Carlo and Italy. Our daughter would be away on her own summer program, and Benny would be at diabetes camp. Little did we know how much problem-solving would come into play.

I've helped out at diabetes camp check-in, and there were always two kinds of parents. The newly diagnosed or new-to-camp parents didn't want to leave and would linger after check-in and talk to staff or volunteers like me. Would their child be safe and happy? Would camp be fun? Diabetes or not, it's hard to leave your child for the first time!

The other type of parents would barely stop the car. "We're off to catch a flight!" they'd say after hugging their happy kids and heading out to the parking lot. Or they'd confide that they were staying home and doing nothing but relaxing. Of course, that first night at home still feels pretty weird without carb counting for dinner or the bedtime BG check. But after the first year, most parents are just fine.

I host a drop-off dinner for parents where we share fun camp stories and reassure newer parents. I also do a coffee for the first day of our local diabetes day camp – it's a long weekend run by the pediatric endocrinologists in town. We drink coffee and promise that their children are doing great. It's a nice excuse to hang out with other parents who have kids with T1D.

During the week-long diabetes sleepaway camp, my husband and I had traveled but not for long and never before out of the country. We knew this trip would require some extra work. Benny's diabetes camp is only six days, and we wanted more time than that to really enjoy the trip and justify the long travel time. A plan came together, but as usual for us, it was a bit of a hodgepodge.

We asked Geoffrey, one of Benny's counselors who's more of a family friend now, if he'd be willing to babysit for two nights before camp and then take Benny to camp with him. He agreed, but unfortunately, he couldn't take Benny to camp. The counselors go up early the day before, and unless they're a family member, they can't bring anyone else along.

Plan B: The counselor would hang out with Benny for the first two nights and then take him to stay with a school friend for the night before camp. These were not "diabetes people," but Benny had spent lots of time at this house and had slept over before. Another friend of mine – a fellow diabetes parent – would pick Benny up on their way to diabetes camp. Lots of moving parts, but we had a plan in place with people I trusted.

We packed three bags: one for the days before camp, one for the week of camp, and the smaller diabetes bag Benny takes most places with all of his medical supplies for the entire length we'd be gone. Our diabetes camp provides insulin, but I always like a backup, so between pens and vials, I threw about a month's worth of insulin into his medical bag.

We waved goodbye and headed to the airport. I admit, I had a moment of panic before we boarded the plane. I'm not a great flyer anyway, but this was the first time I'd left the country without my children. My husband looked at me, close to panic, and said we can do whatever you want. He meant it. He would've sat in that airport and waited for another plane or taken me home. He hugged me, and that's all I needed. I took a deep breath and got on the plane. I knew Benny was in good hands. I knew my daughter was fine. Even so, I ordered a drink right away.

Slade had taken care of our cell phones. We'd have Wi-Fi in hotels, but I wanted to be able to text anytime during our trip. The last time we had done anything with cell phones and international travel was on a cruise; we told everyone to turn off their Wi-Fi, but our daughter didn't fully get it, and left hers on. She played games and used apps for the entire week, and we were hit with a huge bill when we got home. All that Animal Crossing and Candy Crush added up! Somehow my husband was able to talk it down to $60, but we'd learned.

I wasn't planning on watching the Dexcom our entire trip, but it was nice to know it was there. Nothing eventful happened for the first two days, and we had a great time in Monte Carlo. Our first date had been at a casino. Checking out the glamor and glitz of Monaco seemed like an appropriate way to celebrate 20 years together. It did not disappoint.

On the third day, we took a train to Italy, checked in late, and fell into bed. At 2 a.m. my phone buzzed with a text from Benny.

"Mom. I'm really high. Can you help me figure out what to do? We were noodling all day."

Despite living in the south for 20 years, noodling is not something I'm personally familiar with. To be honest, fishing is not something I'm personally familiar with. Noodling is sort of a cousin of fishing. Or maybe more like a weird downstairs neighbor. When one noodles, one is catching catfish. With one's hands.

Earlier that day, Greg's dad had sent us a great picture of the boys grinning, standing behind a pile of catfish. It looked to me like a wall of giant, ugly fish, at least 20, laid out on a long table. The boys looked filthy and happy. Greg's dad had texted it over on his way to bring the boys back to Greg's mom's house, where they'd spend the night.

"Mom. I left my medical bag with all my insulin and everything in Greg's dad's car. I don't have any insulin left in my cartridge, and I'm really high. What do I do?"

Even as my sleepy brain struggled to read the words, my heart sank. We'd talked in advance about taking his medical bag on the fishing trip, but being careful not to leave it in the sun all day, and about not dropping his cell phone in the water. We had not talked about forgetting the bag that held *all* of his insulin.

OK. It was 2 a.m. Deep breath. I texted back that he should wake up Greg's mom and drive to our house, less than ten minutes away. He could go in and get whatever he needed. We had more insulin in the fridge and supplies in our cabinet. I told him to then call me back, and we'd figure out dosing.

"Don't worry about waking up Greg's mom," I texted. "That's what parents do on a sleepover – she'll understand."

"Mom. What are you talking about? It's 8 o'clock here, and

Mrs. M. is right here next to me. Greg's dad is already on his way back with my bag. He dropped me off less than ten minutes ago."

My brain reeled. I looked at my phone. 8 p.m.? It was the middle of the night! But … I had completely forgotten about time zones. And by the frantic tone of that first text, I had assumed Greg's dad was long gone. This just went from a borderline emergency to a walk in the park. Time to switch gears.

"OK," I texted. "Oops. So. What's your plan? You tell me what you should do."

I waited as he typed.

"I'm going to put in a new cartridge and change my inset just in case. I think I'll correct by shot first, then put my pump back on. I also forgot to tell you that my Dexcom came out earlier today. That's why I didn't realize how high I was until we got back to the house." He was over 400.

"Great plan! Since no Dexcom, also set an alarm for three hours after you go to bed. With all that new insulin and such a big high, you might go low. You don't have to text me, but feel free to anytime you have a question or are worried."

"OK, sounds good."

He texted me again when he had the insulin back in hand and had executed the plan he laid out. Everything was settled, and I went back to bed.

Weeks later, at that teen session, I would feel my eyes water when Jill mentioned problem-solving. Benny was doing that. Sure, I had a bunch of people helping out, and yes, he had messed up. But I knew that if he hadn't been able to reach me, he knew how to work out a plan. He would be able to solve these issues.

He also had a backstop of being able to call the camp counselor if he needed to or my diabetes mom friend who was picking him up the next day to go to camp. At the worst, Greg's mom could have called our endo on call.

I was grateful to be there for him and heartened to know this was a good sign. I remember thinking something like, "Well, at least we're getting some things right!"

I don't remember having trouble getting back to sleep in Italy that night. I know that when I woke up, I was itching to find out how the rest of the night had gone. But it was 7 a.m. my time, and only 1 a.m. in North Carolina. Finally, I texted him around 8 a.m. his time. Everything was fine. He had set the alarm and checked BG three hours after bed as we'd discussed.

"I'm not going to tell you how low I was or how much I ate. But I will tell you that Papa John's has a cookie pizza, and it's delicious."

Problem-solving.

ASK YOUR DOCTOR

- If I think my child is ready, what are some safe ways to practice letting them make their own treatment decisions?

- If we run out of insulin (or lose it), what's the best way to get an emergency refill? Is that something you can help us with?

CHAPTER 20

The Pressure
To Be Perfect

Over the years, I've come up with my own
philosophy about Benny's diabetes care: Don't
worry about perfect; go for safe and happy. Do I love
my child? Am I doing my best? Is he happy? Is our
endo happy? Yes. Then let's keep working in the
right direction.

A s I say on the podcast, before I let you go, let's talk about one
more thing.

After reading this book, you know I don't believe in the
pursuit of diabetes perfection. Even so, I'm still surprised at how
many people expect it, who strive for it and feel guilt or shame
because they feel they don't measure up. We were lucky our endo
told us right away that T1D management is just as much art as
science. Over the years, I've come up with my own philosophy
about Benny's diabetes care: Don't worry about perfect; go for
safe and happy. Do I love my child? Am I doing my best? Is he
happy? Is our endo happy? Yes. Then let's keep working in that
right direction.

I've shared that thought with parents who've then burst into
tears. That's not a joke. The realization that a happy, healthy child
is enough can be a revelation.

There is so much pressure right now for straight CGM lines and for amazing A1Cs that I worry we may lose sight that we're raising children, not numbers. My kid is an athlete, a goofball, a friend, a student, a gamer. Not a 6.1 or a 7.5 or a 9.4.

When we share A1Cs or post pictures of flat CGM lines, what's the message? It can be great: "Hey! Look how I'm doing in this hard-fought battle. Celebrate with me!" Or it can be a bit clueless: "Wow, look at my amazing 5-year-old! We've got this figured out forever!" (That was me, by the way. Puberty is a bit humbling.) It can even be dangerous: "Our way is the only way. I don't know anything about you, but if you're not managing my way, you're doing it wrong."

I stopped posting Benny's A1Cs a long time ago, mostly because it's not my information to share, and I don't want to leave a long trail of medical information on the internet. But I also stopped because when I left the actual number out, something amazing happened. More people responded, were encouraging, and shared their own stories and feelings.

Parenting with diabetes is difficult, in part, because parenting is difficult. We all do this in our own way. What works for me may horrify you. Unlike those energetic moms on Pinterest, I will never turn my kids' lunches into works of art. While diabetes parent conversations are less about cutting sandwiches into fancy shapes, there still seems to be a competition over who can out-parent. Night checks, remote monitoring, what pump to use, what to do at school – talking about these issues can sometimes feel like wading into a minefield.

Numbers are a bit easier to focus on. They're less messy than life, more orderly. And technology has brought amazing insight and help into our lives. I wouldn't want to go without the CGM, but in a weird way, I'm grateful we didn't have it for the first seven years of diagnosis. It gave me a more practical perspective and set us up for realistic and effective use. Insulin is so much slower than that real-time BG graph. You need to figure out your child's body and your child's unique diabetes before you freak out about lines and alarms.

If Benny were diagnosed today, I'd want a CGM as soon as possible. But as great as the information is, it can become another point of comparison. What's your high alarm set to? How long can you keep a sensor on? If we can measure it, human nature is to compare and compete. And, for me at least, someone else is always going to be "better."

Do not misunderstand: I would never suggest that people with diabetes can relax or back off managing this crappy condition. It's a lot of hard work all the time. But it's important to acknowledge that even hard work won't make you perfect. In addition to counting carbs, eating mindfully, bolusing appropriately, and setting good basal rates, we all know we're supposed to eat well, exercise, sleep enough, and lower our stress. I'm coming up short on most of those, and I don't even have diabetes!

The best advice a doctor ever gave me is, "Be kind to yourself." We all need to work harder on that. Love and treasure your child with T1D, and be kind to yourself. Back off the pressure to be perfect and start enjoying the safe and happy.

ASK YOUR DOCTOR

- Can you explain how timing of our type of insulin works, particularly how it seems to work for my child? Do we need to adjust any settings, such as insulin-on-board (IOB), if using an insulin pump?

- What are our long-term goals with type 1 diabetes? Beyond A1C, can you help me zoom out and think about my child's overall well-being?

- What do you think is the best way to use a CGM to maximum physical and mental benefit?

Acknowledgments

I'm grateful to so many who helped bring this book to life. Thanks to everyone mentioned in my stories. Living as a family with type 1 diabetes on board is a long and challenging journey, and we've been incredibly fortunate to find people willing to walk this path with us. Thank you for making our road a little bit smoother.

I want to acknowledge a few people in the diabetes online community (DOC) who helped me early on and continue to guide me today. Kerri Sparling, Scott Johnson, Cherise Shockley, and Christel Marchand Aprigliano shared their real-life stories about living with type 1 diabetes in a way that spoke to me. More wonderful writers and storytellers continue to join our community, but the words I read in the first weeks and months after Benny's diagnosis made an indelible impression and guided our T1D management from the start.

For parenting advice, I can't thank Moira McCarthy enough. Moira is a wonderful writer, a dear friend, and now my fellow "dope D-mom" on the "Diabetes Connections" podcast. When I was reading her blog back in 2007, I never thought she'd be the first reader of samples that became this book. I also want to thank other diabetes mom friends like Anne Sutton and Tina Ghosn who know sharing the not-so-perfect is where the most meaningful connections and support happen.

Thanks to my podcast listeners who have created their own community within the DOC. I hope the stories I share on the show help you in the same way those early blogs and posts helped us.

Thanks to Linnet for behind-the-scenes support throughout this project and, of course, for being our partner in diabetes management since before Benny could say those words. She is part of our incredible care team that includes Dr. V and our local pediatric endo practice. We are so fortunate that the health care providers we met on day one were the right match for us.

Thanks to everyone at SPARK Publications for believing in this project. Some days, I think Larry Preslar believed in it more than I did! Thanks to Mel Graham for keeping me on task with those pesky deadlines and to Jim Denk for that fantastic cover illustration. Thanks, especially, to Fabi Preslar for her guidance and wisdom.

Thank you to my sister, Melissa, and my mom, Arlene, for your help on this book and, more importantly, for living this life with us. You are always there to listen when I question my decisions, need to rant and rave about diabetes, or simply need to cry. We somehow always find the laughter together. Thanks, too, for reading early versions of the book and being honest with criticism and feedback. To have you both cheering me on during this process was a gift.

A huge thank you to Lea and Benny for giving me permission to share these stories in the hopes that someone else will learn from our mistakes. When I first broached the subject, I was told these stories only make me look bad. I can live with that!

Finally, thanks to Slade for encouraging me and standing by my side every step of the way. Who knew the 1995 Utica Saint Patrick's Day Parade would start my life's great adventure: my family with you.

About the Author

Stacey Simms hosts the award-winning podcast "Diabetes Connections." Her son was diagnosed with type 1 diabetes (T1D) in 2006, one month before he turned 2 years old, and Stacey started blogging about her family's experience with T1D a few weeks later. For more than a decade, she hosted "Charlotte's Morning News" on WBT-AM, the city's top-rated morning radio news show. Stacey has been named to Diabetes Forecast magazine's People to Know, the Charlotte Business Journal's 40 Under 40, and Mecklenburg Times' 50 Most Influential Women. She lives near Charlotte, North Carolina, with her husband, two children, and their dog, Freckles.

CONNECT WITH STACEY ONLINE

- diabetes-connections.com
- staceysimms.com
- staceyrsimms
- staceysimms
- staceysimms

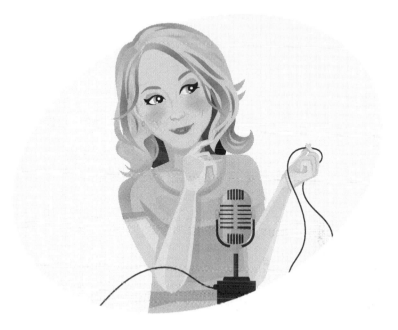

diabetes-connections.com

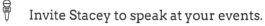
Listen to the podcast.

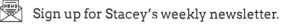
Sign up for Stacey's weekly newsletter.

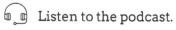
Invite Stacey to speak at your events.

Made in the USA
Middletown, DE
15 November 2020